# The Skin Care Answer Book

## Real-World Answers to 275 Most-Asked Skin Care Questions

Mark Lees, Ph.D.

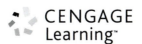
CENGAGE
Learning™

Australia • Brazil • Japan • Korea • Mexico • Singapore • Spain • United Kingdom • United States

FEB 2010

Hu

# CENGAGE Learning™

**The Skin Care Answer Book,
First Edition
Mark Lees**

President, Milady: Dawn Gerrain

Publisher: Erin O'Connor

Acquisitions Editor: Martine Edwards

Senior Product Manager: Philip Mandl

Editorial Assistant: Elizabeth Edwards

Director of Beauty Industry Relations:
Sandra Bruce

Senior Marketing Manager:
Gerard McAvey

Marketing Coordinator: Matt McGuire

Production Director: Wendy Troeger

Senior Content Project Manager:
Nina Tucciarelli

Manufacturing Buyer: Charlene Taylor

Senior Art Director: Joy Kocsis

Content Project Management:
Pre-PressPMG

Compositor: Pre-PressPMG

Cover Design: MW Design

Cover Images: © Shutterstock images

For product information and technology assistance, contact us at
**Professional & Career Group Customer Support, 1-800-648-7450**

For permission to use material from this text or product,
submit all requests online at **cengage.com/permissions**
Further permissions questions can be emailed to
**permissionrequest@cengage.com**

Library of Congress Control Number: 2009934804

ISBN-13: 978-1-4354-8225-8

ISBN-10: 1-4354-8225-5

**Milady**
5 Maxwell Drive
Clifton Park, NY 12065-2919
USA

Cengage Learning products are represented in Canada by Nelson Education, Ltd.

For your lifelong learning solutions, visit **milady.cengage.com**

Visit our corporate website at **cengage.com**

Printed in the United States of America
1 2 3 4 5 XX 14 13 12 11 10

*This book is dedicated to my mother,*
*Dr. Virginia Lees. Thank you for your teaching*
*and communication skills!*

# CONTENTS

## 3. Acne and Acne-Prone Skin   49

## 5. Dry Skin 103

## 6. Sun Care 119

## 10. Problems That Need a Doctor    195

# ABOUT THE AUTHOR

Dr. Mark Lees is one of the country's most noted skin care specialists, an award-winning speaker and product developer, and has been actively practicing clinical skin care for over 20 years at his multi-award-winning CIDESCO accredited Florida salon, which has won multiple awards for "Best Facial," "Best Massage," and "Best Pampering Place" by the readers of the *Pensacola News-Journal*.

His professional awards are numerous and include American Salon Magazine Esthetician of the Year, the Les Nouvelles Esthetiques Crystal Award, the Dermascope Legends Award, the Rocco Bellino Award for outstanding education from the Chicago Cosmetology Association, and Best Educational Skin Care Classroom from the Long Beach International Beauty Expo. Dr. Lees has also been inducted into the National Cosmetology Association's Hall of Renown.

Dr. Lees has been interviewed and quoted by NBC News, The Associated Press, the Discovery Channel, *Glamour*, *Self*, *Teen*, *Shape Magazine*, and many other publications.

Dr. Lees is cofounder of the Institute of Advanced Clinical Esthetics in Seattle, special science-based advanced training programs for clinical estheticians.

Dr. Lees is former chairman of EstheticsAmerica, the esthetics education division of the National Cosmetology Association, and has served as a CIDESCO International Examiner. He has also served on the national Board of Directors of the NCA.

Dr. Lees is former chairman of the board of the Esthetics Manufacturers and Distributors Alliance, is a member of the Society of Cosmetic Chemists, and is author of the popular book **Skin Care: Beyond the Basics**, now in its third edition, and contributing science author of **Milady' Comprehensive Training for Estheticians**. He holds a Ph.D. in Health Sciences, a Master of Science in Health, and a CIDESCO International Diploma. He is licensed to practice in both Florida and Washington State. His line of products for problem, sensitive, and sun-damaged skin is available at finer salons and clinics throughout the United States.

# ACKNOWLEDGMENTS

Very special thanks to the following people and organizations for contributing in many ways to this book. The author appreciates their efforts.

Martine Edwards, Philip Mandl, and all the team at Milady/Cengage Learning

My incredible team at Mark Lees Skin Care

My wonderful family and friends

Reviewers:

Sophia Camejo, Tarzana, California

Dayspa Magazine, Van Nuys, California

Dermascope Magazine, Garland, Texas

Rebecca James-Gadberry, Instructor of Cosmetic Science, UCLA Extension, Los Angeles, California

Derek Jones, M.D., Facial Plastic Surgeon, Pensacola, Florida

Les Nouvelles Esthetiques—American Edition, Coral Gables, Florida

Anne Martin, Seattle, Washington

Howard Murad, M.D., Dermatologist, Murad, Inc., Los Angeles, California

Peter Pugliese, M.D., Circadia by Dr. Pugliese; Bernville, Pennsylvania

Revitalight; Chicago, Illinois

Skin, Inc., Carol Stream, Illinois

David Suzuki, Bio-Therapeutic, Inc., Seattle, Washington

# FOREWORD

**Howard Murad, M.D.**

Perhaps it is a dermatologist's bias, but I am often amazed by how little the average person knows about skin. This complex and remarkable fabric is the body's largest, most visible, and in many ways most vulnerable organ.

In *The Skin Care Answer Book*, Dr. Mark Lees has taken on the enormous challenge of explaining the structure and function of skin, as well as the pathology, symptomatology, and treatment of common skin disorders in terms that both laypeople and skin care professionals can understand. The resulting volume is a clear and concise guide that will make a great contribution to the educational goals of the skin care industry—and will help clear up some culturally ingrained misperceptions about skin and its care.

In my work as a doctor, a professor, and founder of one of America's leading clinical skin care companies, I have met and collaborated with countless people in the world of skin care, yet few have made the kind of impression on me that Dr. Mark Lees has. There are so many ways in which Dr. Lees has distinguished himself—as a skin care professional, skin care products developer, scholar, educator, author, and industry leader. In each realm, Dr. Lees has focused his intelligence, passion, and creativity to accomplish the extraordinary.

Given Mark's exceptional background, it is no surprise that *The Skin Care Answer Book* is a thoughtful, well-researched, and comprehensive treatment of issues related to skin and skin health as well as a user-friendly guide that invites exploration and holds the reader's attention.

That a guide with the sophistication of *The Skin Care Answer Book* is designed to be used as a reference for esthetics professionals and consumers reminds us of how far the world of esthetics has come and of the many ways that barriers between medical and esthetic care have fallen by the wayside. In many ways, both Dr. Lees and I were pioneering advocates for these changes, and our collaborations over the years are prime examples of what can be accomplished when skin care professionals can acknowledge the unique contributions that different disciplines can make.

I first met Dr. Lees when I was launching Murad Skin care. Even though Dr. Lees had his own line of products, he was willing to hear me out and let me demonstrate the unique benefits of my revolutionary AHA treatments. I could tell we were kindred spirits by his eagerness to start using the products in his spa immediately. Like me, Dr. Lees was excited to discover something new that could help his clients and wasn't going to let ego or economics get in the way.

What the reader will find embodied in these pages, and in Dr. Lees himself, is a passion for education that is rooted in a broader passion for helping people have the healthy, vibrant skin that they desire and deserve. That passion is the force that animates the day-to-day operation of his flagship spa, his countless appearances on television and in print, his educational efforts, and his own line of skin care products. Since that same passion for skin health has defined my remarkably rewarding journey, perhaps there is something to be said for putting people before profits as a strategy for success in the world of skin care.

I share Dr. Lees' fundamental belief that our industry will continue to prosper as long as we continue our commitment to taking care of the unique needs of each individual, work hard to advance the level of professionalism, and remember that the skin is not only the body's largest organ—it is the body's most interconnected organ and a therapeutic gateway to a world of wellness.

Regardless of whether one is looking for a primer on skin care or a ready reference for use as questions arise, *The Skin Care Answer Book* is a must-have volume that reflects the innovative thinking of one of America's most widely regarded authorities on skin and esthetical care.

**Howard Murad, M.D., is an associate clinical professor of dermatology at UCLA, founder of Murad Skincare, Inc., the pioneering researcher who unlocked the secrets of The Science of Cellular Water, and the author of the Inclusive Health philosophy.**

# LETTER TO THE READER

Since the early 1990s, skin care has become a true science, with many effective topical treatments that change the skin's appearance. Many of these treatments were only dreamed about prior to this era.

In addition, we are living in the information age, where information is as close as any computer. Unfortunately, there is also much misinformation available online. Rumors and erroneous information abound, and there is a real need to sort the facts. In almost three decades of practice as a clinical skin therapist and skin care product developer, I have had thousands of questions posed to me. There are, however, many questions that I answer over and over.

*The Skin Care Answer Book* provides the answers to almost 300 of the most-asked skin care questions, plus advice as to when to seek the help of a medical professional. It is a question-and-answer book written for consumers but also can be used by practicing estheticians, skin therapists, dermatology nurses, and skin care educators for quick reference.

Many clients have more than one problem with their skin. I hope that this book will provide good and easy-to-understand information to help them find an answer for their problems. I also hope that it will help everyone have more beautiful and healthy skin for a lifetime.

**Mark Lees, Ph.D., M.S.**
CIDESCO Diplomate

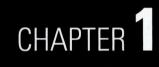

# CHAPTER 1

# Understanding the Skin

**Q** **Is the outside of the skin really dead?**

**A** Technically, yes, at least for most of the outermost layer of the skin. However, this outermost layer of the skin, the **epidermis,** is the first line of defense against dehydration, bacterial invasion, and irritant penetration. You can think of the epidermis as the outside wall of a fort. It is this layer that we take care of when we practice a skin care program.

The cells in the epidermis go through many biochemical changes, and there are many functions of this layer even though most of it is technically dead.

There are three types of active cells in the epidermis: the **basal cells,** the **melanocytes,** and the **Langerhans cells.**

- The melanocytes are the pigment-producing cells that are found in both the lower epidermis and the dermis. Melanocytes give skin its color and are responsible for tanning.
- The Langerhans cells are immune function cells that "patrol" the epidermis to detect foreign invaders or pathogens.
- The basal cells, described in more detail below, are the cells that make new skin cells in the epidermis.

**Q** **How does the skin renew itself?**

**A** The cells in the outer layer of the skin, the epidermis, begin as live cells in the lowest layer of the epidermis known as the **basal layer.** The basal layer used to be called the *germinative layer* or the *stratum germinativum*.

The basal cells divide in a biological process called **mitotic division,** forming new, identical cells. These fresh cells are pushed upward due to the mitotic division and begin their journey toward the outside surface of the skin. As they approach the surface, these cells are going through a process called **keratinization.**

During this process, the cells fill with a protein called **keratin.** There are two types of keratin. The type in the epidermal skin cells is soft keratin, which is the same type that is in hair. Hard keratin is present in the fingernails and toenails and gives the strength and ridged feel to these structures. Keratin's main structure in the skin is to make the skin surface more resilient and resistant to water absorption/evaporation; to resist invasion by foreign substances or organisms, such as bacteria; and to help keep the skin from becoming dry and dehydrated.

During the process of the cells moving from the innermost to the outermost layers of the epidermis, these cells change shape several times and go through several named layers within the epidermis. While in each layer, there are more biochemical changes happening to these epidermal cells.

After leaving the basal layer in their journey toward the skin surface, the cells begin to flatten out and form a layer called the **spiny layer** or **stratum spinosum.** From this layer they move farther upward into a layer called the **granular layer** or **stratum granulosum,** where the cells look "grainy" because they are beginning to be filled with keratin. The last and outermost layer in the epidermis is the **stratum corneum,** also called the *horny layer* due to their appearance under a microscope. The cells in the corneum are much flatter and stacked liked shingles on a roof.

All of the cells going through the process of keratinization are referred to often as **keratinocytes.** This is a general term to describe cells in the epidermis, regardless of layer or stage of the process. Keratinocytes that are specifically in the stratum corneum are called **corneocytes.**

A good analogy for the keratinization process is the transformation of a grape into a raisin. Like a grape, the basal cells are fresh, rounded, and plump. As the grape ages and dries, the structure becomes dehydrated, with hardened denser fibers, and is more resilient and harder. The raisin represents the corneocyte, stacked like shingles on a roof on the surface of the skin, providing the first line of protection for the skin, preventing penetration of possible harmful or inflammatory substances, and preventing water loss that results in dehydration.

**Q** **Is any part of the skin alive?**

**A** Yes. We have just discussed the epidermis, containing mostly dead or dying cells, but we have also learned how active this layer is biologically.

The skin is actually the largest organ in the human body! The **dermis** of the skin is the layer under the epidermis and is very much alive. The differences between the live layer and dead/dying layers of the skin are as follows:

- The live layer contains blood and blood vessels. The epidermis does not.
- The live layer contains nerve endings that sense heat, cold, pain, pressure, and touch.
- The epidermis sheds and renews itself constantly. The dermis does not shed or have a renewal cycle.

The dermis contains the collagen, elastin, and other support substances that give the skin its structure and form. The dermis also contains blood vessels to nourish the many active and different living cells in this area. These include both arteries and veins. Arteries carry blood to the tissues, and veins return deoxygenated blood to the heart and lungs for reoxygenation.

The dermis is made up of two major layers. The **papillary dermis** is at the top of the dermis and connects the dermis to the epidermis. This attachment point is known as the **epidermal-dermal junction.** The papillary dermis contains many blood capillaries and nerves that are sensitive to the touch. The papillary dermis also contains melanocytes, which are the pigment-producing cells that give skin its color and that are also responsible for tanning.

The **reticular dermis** is the lower and thicker part of the dermis. The reticular dermis contains **collagen** that gives firmness to the skin and **elastin** that gives flexibility and elasticity to the skin. These protein fibers run throughout the reticular dermis.

A filler-like substance called **ground substance** fills empty spaces in the reticular dermis. This jellylike substance is made of water-binding biochemicals such as **glycosaminoglycans,** which hold tremendous amounts of water. **Hyaluronic acid** is an ingredient well known in moisturizers which holds 1,000 times its own weight in water. Hyaluronic acid is a component within the ground substance. Unfortunately, the hyaluronic acid in moisturizers is a large molecule that cannot penetrate the skin or replace dermal ground substance. It can only work on the surface as a water-binder.

Running from the base of the reticular dermis through the papillary layer and the epidermis are the ducts of the sebaceous and sweat glands.

The reticular layer also contains more sensory nerve endings and larger blood vessels that feed the capillaries in the papillary dermis.

The **sebaceous glands,** the **sudoriferous** (sweat) **glands,** and the base of the hair **follicle** are all in the reticular layer.

Beneath the reticular dermis is another layer called the **subcutaneous layer,** which contains thicker layers of fat to give the skin protection and to cushion the internal organs. This fat also helps with temperature regulation and insulates the blood vessels and nerve fibers that are also running through this layer.

**Q** So, how many layers are there in the skin?

**A** There are three main layers: the epidermis, the dermis, and the subcutaneous layer.

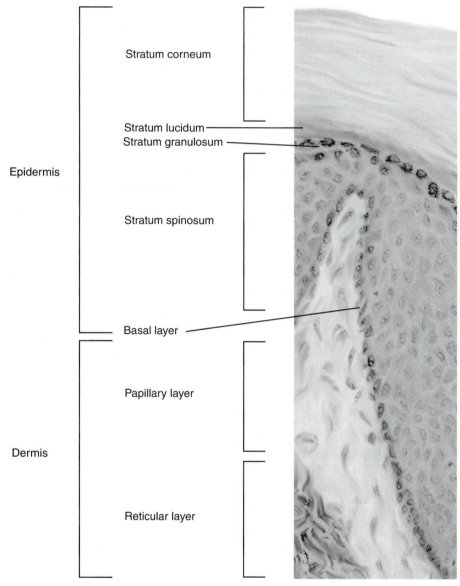

Epidermis

Stratum corneum

Stratum lucidum
Stratum granulosum

Stratum spinosum

Basal layer

Dermis

Papillary layer

Reticular layer

The layers and sublayers of the skin.

The epidermis has four or five layers, depending on the area of the body:

- The basal layer, where the cells divide, and also where melanocytes are present
- The spinosum or "prickle" layer, just above the basal layer where the keratinization process is beginning

- The granular layer that contains grainy-looking cells containing the **lamellar bodies** that produce lipids for the barrier function, the complex of lipids within the epidermis that helps protect the skin from dehydration and irritant invasion
- The corneum, the outermost layer of the epidermis—the shingles on the roof
- The stratum lucidum, an additional layer, also sometimes called the "clear layer," that is between the granular and corneum layers and is only found in the skin of the soles of the feet and palms of the hands.

The dermis contains two main layers:

- The papillary dermis, which attaches to the epidermis, and is therefore the outermost layer of the dermis
- The reticular dermis, the lower layer in the dermis, containing blood vessels, nerve endings, collagen, and elastin fibers.

The subcutaneous layer is located under the dermis and is a fatty layer that provides structure and cushion for the skin.

**Q** **How thick is the skin?**

**A** This depends on the area of the body. Generally the skin is between 1 millimeter and 5 millimeters thick. The soles of the feet have the thickest skin. The eyelid skin is the thinnest.

The epidermis is very thin. If you have ever had a paper cut, you will know how thin the epidermis is. Remember, there is no blood in the epidermis, so when the skin bleeds, the injury has gone through the epidermis and into the dermis.

**Q** **Why does skin get dry and chapped?**

**A** Exposure to the elements, especially in extreme temperatures, causes water in the skin surface to evaporate, drying the surface and eventually causing enough damage to produce chapping. The barrier function of the skin is severely damaged in chapped skin.

**Q** **What does *barrier function* mean?**

**A** **Barrier function** refers to the complex of lipids (fatty materials such as ceramides, fatty acids, and cholesterol) that is present between the cells in the corneum. This lipid barrier guards moisture (transepidermal water loss, or TEWL) and protects against dehydration, and it also provides a lipid barrier to prevent irritants from entering the skin. If you think of the epidermis as a brick wall, the cells are the bricks and are held together by the mortar that is the barrier lipid complex, sometimes also referred to as the **intercellular lipid matrix** or **intercellular cement.** The lipids fill in the gaps between the cells in the same way mortar fills the spaces between bricks in a wall.

If you have ever accidentally dripped lemon juice on a chapped place on your hand, you will understand how the barrier lipid complex (or lack of it, as in chapped skin) protects the skin. When the skin is chapped, it has lost lipids in the barrier function, easily allowing the penetration of

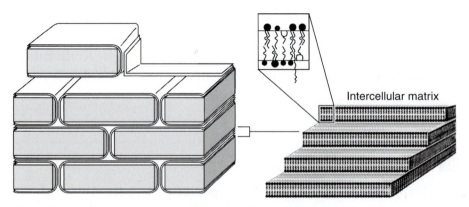

Intercellular matrix

The "brick and mortar" concept of the skin's barrier function.

irritants such as lemon juice. When the acidic lemon juice hits a nerve ending, it stings and burns.

When the barrier function is fully intact, lemon juice or most irritants cannot easily penetrate the skin surface. Likewise, the skin cannot lose water and become dehydrated when the barrier is intact.

**Q** How does the barrier function form?

**A** The barrier function lipids are formed during the keratinization process. Beginning in the spinosum, structures within the cells that are keratinizing, called lamellar bodies, begin forming. These lamellar bodies eventually produce the lipid complex that over time fills the gaps between the cells in the stratum corneum.

**Q** What can damage the barrier function?

**A** Exposure to elements, especially cold, heat, dry air, and wind, can damage the lipids in the barrier. Sun exposure certainly can also cause an impaired barrier. Skin that is unprotected in the winter will have a strong tendency to become dehydrated due to the destruction of barrier lipids.

Overcleansing or using soaps or cleansers that are too strong for the skin type can damage the barrier. Using or overusing high-foaming detergent cleansers can strip the skin of protective sebum, and it then begins slowly stripping the fats within the barrier function.

Likewise, over-exfoliation can strip too many surface corneum cells and along with these cells, the barrier lipids are also depleted.

Sun and exposure to cold, low humidity, or wind can also severely impair the barrier. Cumulative sun damage can severely affect the cell renewal cycle, which is how the lipids are naturally formed.

When the barrier function is damaged, it is said to be **impaired.**

**Q.** What are the symptoms of impaired barrier function?

**A.** There are many symptoms of impaired barrier function, and they may vary with the skin type, severity of impairment, and other related skin conditions. For example, people who have rosacea often have skin barrier impairment problems.

Impaired barrier function can affect sensitivity, inflammation, skin dryness, hyperpigmentation from inflammation, and aging symptoms.

Some of the common symptoms of an impaired barrier function may be the following:

- Flaking—A typical sign of dehydrated skin.
- Tightness—A sensation that occurs when the barrier has been damaged, such as the feeling of tightness of the body skin that may be experienced after a soapy or hot bath.
- Redness—Inflammation that often occurs because the barrier is unable to protect against irritants penetrating the skin.
- Itchiness—**Winter itch** is classic barrier function damage. The damaged barrier function affects nerve endings, causing itching. When the dehydrated skin is scratched to relieve the itching, the barrier function may be further injured, and inflammation and redness can result or worsen.
- Stinging—Stinging may result from irritants easily penetrating the skin and inflaming the nerve endings.

**Q.** Does the barrier function affect the esthetic appearance of the skin?

**A.** Yes! If the barrier is fully intact and healthy, the skin will hold moisture well, which makes skin look more supple, firmer, and younger.

Impaired barrier function can make skin look chapped and more wrinkled with many fine lines, and reflect light abnormally. Deep wrinkles and expression lines are accentuated. Skin with poor barrier function is often said to look somewhat "deflated."

Impaired barrier function can also lead to redness due to irritant reactions. The redness associated with rosacea and sensitive skin is often related to impaired barrier function.

**Q** Can the barrier function be improved?

**A** Yes. Using protective emollient products, such as a good moisturizer with emollient protectants such as silicone or petrolatum, will not only protect the barrier from damage, but it will also allow the skin to repair the damaged barrier lipid layer through the cell renewal process.

Products that contain lipid components can help to supplement the missing lipids in damaged skin. For much more on treating dry skin and barrier damage see Chapter 5.

**Q** Why does the skin make oil (sebum)?

**A** Deep in the reticular dermis, near the bottom of the hair follicle, are the sebaceous glands, which secrete (produce) **sebum,** a complex of oily and waxy components. The sebum exits to the surface of the skin via the follicle canal. The entire structure of the follicle is called the **pilosebaceous unit**.

The purpose of sebum is controversial. Some scientists think that it is secreted as an additional surface barrier to help prevent dehydration of the skin. Some think it is a leftover from human evolution. Some think that it has no real purpose. What is known is that skin that is *alipidic* (does not produce much sebum) has a strong tendency to become dehydrated, which supports the first theory.

**Q** Why does the skin have pores?

**A** **Pores** are simply openings or orifices of the sebaceous follicles on the surface of the skin. The pore is not the entire structure, just the opening itself.

**Q** **Why do some people have bigger pores than others?**

**A** The size of the pore is determined by the amount of sebum being produced and flowing down the follicular canal. The more sebum produced, the more the follicle and pore stretch to accommodate the quantity of sebum being secreted. Follicles that are clogged with keratinized cells and fatty materials will have larger pores due to the stretching of the follicle walls from the amount of debris in the canal.

**Q** **Is there a difference between facial and body skin?**

**A** Yes, there many differences, and there are even differences in the skin in different areas of the body:

- There are more sebaceous glands on the face, but there also lots of sebaceous glands in the skin on the scalp, chest, and back. Anywhere there is hair, there are sebaceous glands.
- The sweat glands are more numerous in the palms of the hands and soles of the feet than anywhere else in the body's skin.
- The skin on the face tends to be more sensitive and reactive than body skin.
- The muscles under the facial skin are attached to the skin so that facial expressions can be made. You cannot make expressions with your arm!
- Body skin tends to be drier than facial skin. Perhaps this is because there are fewer sebaceous glands on the body, or perhaps it is because people generally take better care of their facial skin than they do their body skin.
- Acne most often occurs on the face but can also affect the chest, scalp, back, and even the legs.

**Q** **Are there differences between male and female skin?**

**A** There are many differences between male and female skin, but most are due to hormones, not actual anatomical differences.

It is often hard to look at the face of an infant and know if the child is a boy or a girl. This certainly changes at puberty, and puberty is when the sex hormones begin producing the adult sex characteristics of women and men.

The beard skin of a man, male pattern baldness, active sebaceous glands, and body hair growth and type are a few examples of these hormonal differences. These characteristics are all typical of androgenic (male hormone) activity. The soft skin of a woman, the fact that women have more glycosaminoglycans in their reticular dermis, and more fat in the subcutaneous layer is also hormonally related, specifically to estrogen and female hormones.

There are abnormalities in hormone activity that can cause females to grow facial hair or lose scalp hair in a typical male pattern. In females, chronic chin acne and melasma (pregnancy mask) and other pigmentary problems are examples of hormone abnormalities that may require medical treatment to correct. Men rarely have melasma, and men can lose body hair from hormonal problems.

Esthetically, men's skin tends to be oilier than women's and less likely to become dehydrated. Some differences in male and female esthetic skin issues, such as cellulite and lip wrinkling, are related to both hormonal factors and underlying muscle structure differences between the sexes. Women, percentage-wise, have much more body fat than men.

Men generally do not need as much emollient in their treatment as women and also prefer the feel of a lighter-weight product. Women are more likely to have rosacea, but men are more likely to have phymatous rosacea, the type in which the nose becomes bulbous and the cartilage grows. Sensitive skin is more prevalent in females in general, possibly due to some women's tendency to overtreat the skin, causing barrier function damage.

**Q** Why does the skin get hot and cold?

**A** Temperature regulation is one of the amazing major functions of the skin. Sensory nerves in the skin detect outside heat and cold.

Blood vessels can dilate to pump blood to the skin when the body is overheated, so the blood is closer to the outside of the body and can cool. Sweat is produced by the sudoriferous (sweat) glands, and the evaporation of the sweat cools the skin temperature. Coolness of the skin can be caused by exposure to cold external temperatures, but it also can be caused by reduced blood flow to the skin. That someone may look pale when they are ill shows a reduced skin blood flow at that time. The blood flow is reduced when the body is cold to prevent heat from escaping the body.

**Q** Why does the skin tan?

**A** Melanocytes are cells that produce the skin pigment **melanin,** the material that causes a tan. Melanocytes are mainly located in the basal layer of the epidermis, but they are also in the papillary dermis. In the basal cell layer, melanocytes make up approximately 10% of the cells present. In some darker skin colors, the melanocytes may also be present in the reticular (lower layer) dermis.

Melanocytes produce granules of pigment called **melanosomes.** The melanosomes contain the actual melanin pigment.

Melanocytes are **dendritic** cells, which means they have tentacle-like branches. These branches or **dendrites** enable the melanocytes to "inject" keratinocytes with melanosomes, which gives the skin color, as well as cause a tan.

When the skin is exposed to sun, melanocytes produce pigment as a defense mechanism to shield the cells from damaging UV rays. The melanosome granules produced by the melanocytes after sun exposure are deposited in the skin directly over the nucleus of the cell. So, a tan may look attractive to some people, but it is actually an immune function!

**Q** **Why are there so many skin colors?**

**A** Skin color is mainly determined by genetic factors we receive from our parents. We inherit the amounts of pigment produced by our individual melanocytes. In skin of color, the melanosomes produced by the melanocytes are much larger. The large melanosomes in black skin are deposited in keratinocytes as large, single melanosomes. In Caucasian skin there are multiple smaller melanosomes in each keratinocyte.

The variety of shades in skin of color has to do with the size of the melanosomes produced by the melanocytes. The color is determined by genetic factors that dictate the mix and amount of melanin produced.

There are two basic types of melanin. **Eumelanin** is a brown-black melanin found in darker skin types and also in black or brown hair. **Pheomelanin** is a red-yellow pigment and is found in red hair. Large melanosomes of eumelanin singly deposited in keratinocytes will absorb a lot of light, making the skin appear darker. Smaller melanosomes absorb less light, allowing skin and hair to reflect more light, and appear lighter in color.

Other factors in the skin that affect skin color are redness due to (arterial) red hemoglobin carrying oxygen in the blood, which may be close to the skin surface in lighter (Fitzpatrick I and II) skin types. The low levels of melanin in these skin types combine with the close blood vessels to produce a redder skin color.

Blue tones in the skin are caused by hemoglobin that is not oxygenated. In other words, this is venous (in the veins) hemoglobin returning to the heart and lungs for more oxygen.

Yellow pigments called **carotenoids** are from certain foods we eat, such as carrots, that contain this pigment.

The blend of the blue, red, yellow, and the brown coloring from eumelanin mix to an innumerable variety of skin colors and shades.

**Q** **What is collagen and where does it come from?**

**A** Collagen is a protein that is present in the skin in the form of fibers. It is responsible for skin firmness and youthful-looking skin texture. Skin that has been cumulatively sun-damaged has damaged collagen, which results in the appearance of wrinkles and poor skin texture.

Collagen is found in the lower part of the dermis. There are several types of collagen in the skin. If you removed all the water from the skin, collagen would be 70% of what was left. It is a major component of the skin.

Collagen is produced by specialized cells called **fibroblasts**. Fibroblasts are present in the reticular dermis and produce collagen in the form of chain molecules that look like spiral strings that form a braid-like structure. Collagen is produced by the fibroblasts as three chains that eventually intertwine in a ropelike braid called a **helix**.

Creams that contain collagen cannot replace damaged dermal collagen. Collagen present in creams simply helps to bind water to the skin surface. The molecules of collagen are too large to penetrate through the skin. Fibroblasts present in the dermis can be stimulated to produce more collagen by certain ingredients such as tretinoin (Retin-A or Renova), long-term use of alpha hydroxy acids, peptides, or botanical stimulant ingredients such as plant extracts *Centella asiatica* and *Echinacea angustifolia*.

Daily use of broad-spectrum sunscreens is the most effective treatment for maintaining quality collagen, as the fibroblasts are protected by UVA sunscreen components such as avobenzone, emcamsule, titanium dioxide, or zinc oxide that stop the deep dermal penetration of UVA.

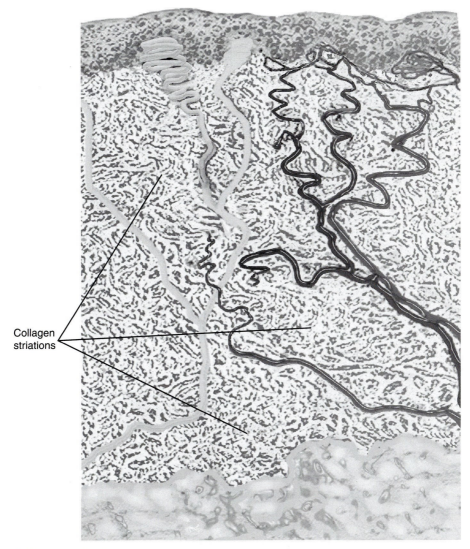

Collagen
striations

Collagen in the dermis.

**Q** **What is the difference between elastin and collagen?**

**A** Collagen and elastin are both protein-based fiber chains present in the dermis. Esthetically, collagen is responsible for skin firmness and turgor, and elastin is responsible for the ability of the skin to stretch and return to its original form.

Estheticians and dermatologists often gently pinch the skin of a client to observe how quickly the skin returns to its original contour to test skin elasticity. If the "return to normal" takes more than a split second, the skin has damaged elastin fibrils. Like collagen, elastin is produced by the fibroblast cells, but unlike collagen it is produced as two intertwined molecules.

Collagen protein is abundant in the skin dermis, while elastin only comprises a small portion of the reticular dermis.

Elastin fibers are found in the upper dermis, unlike collagen, which is found in the lower dermis. Both the collagen and elastin fibrils are surrounded by ground substance. The ground substance is a gel-like substance comprised of large sugar-related molecules called glycosaminoglycans. These molecules include hyaluronic acid, an extremely strong water-binding molecule.

There is not much known about elastin, but more research is being conducted. At this point, there is only one type of elastin known. Elastin is so important for skin elasticity and aging-skin treatment.

As discussed previously, collagen is fairly easy to produce and helps repair the skin esthetically. Elastin is much harder to stimulate. Micro-current has been shown to stimulate elastin production, and it is believed that some of the same stimulants used for collagen production may help stimulate elastin.

**Q** **How does the skin heal after a cut?**

**A** When the skin is injured, a flood of biochemical reactions take place involving the immune system, the blood, and the fibroblasts. The entire biological process of healing is both complicated and amazing. Here we will give a brief overview of how the many systems of the body and different cells types work together to heal a wound.

In a cut, clotting factors in the blood stop the immediate flow of blood from the injury. The immune system is alerted, sending leucocytes (white blood cells) to the area to help fight off any possible infection. The fibroblasts from surrounding tissues migrate to the area of injury and begin producing large amounts of collagen to help rebuild the tissue in the injured area. A "scaffolding" is established at first. Eventually the collagen fills in the separated area in the cut.

Small blood vessels begin to form from larger vessels to help bring more blood to the healing area. Blood flow to the area is a crucial part of wound healing; without it, the cells are not provided with many factors that help with wound healing, including transport of immune cells to fight and prevent infection.

The epidermis is regenerated in a process called **re-epithelialization.** Cells that line the follicle walls in the lower part of the reticular dermis begin replicating. These new cells migrate to the surface via the follicle and begin the formation of the epidermal layers. This is also how the skin heals after resurfacing laser treatment or a deep surgical chemical peel.

Wounds heal better when they are kept moist; they are also less likely to form scars. They should be cleaned daily with fresh water, and an antibiotic ointment should be used. Use of an emollient such as petrolatum (petroleum jelly) keeps the wound moist for better healing.

**Q** Why does the skin sometimes scar after an injury?

**A** The skin quickly forms fibers to bridge the gap in a cut or injury. These collagen fibers are granular-like to fill in where cells are missing. They are fibers, not cells, and have a different texture than the original tissue.

Over time these collagen fibers will soften and the skin tissue will regain much of its original organization in terms of blood vessels and normal skin function.

It can take up to a year for a scar to soften and become flatter. As the area returns to normal, blood flow is normalized, which makes the scar that is a few months old look less red. As collagen fibers reorganize in the healed cut, the scar will flatten out.

Raised scars are referred to as **hypertrophic,** and depressed (sunken) scars, which often are called pockmarks, are known as **hypotrophic.**

Hypertrophic scars resolve and become flatter over time as the skin makes an enzyme called **collagenase,** which breaks up excess collagen in the scar, causing a flattening effect. A **keloid** is a hypertrophic scar that does not resolve because the skin hereditarily does not make collagen in a normal way. Keloids require careful and immediate dermatological treatment with steroid injections to help them reduce in size and elevation. Keloid formation is prevalent in skin of color.

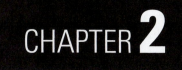

CHAPTER **2**

# Aging and Photo-Aging Skin

21

**Q** What actually causes wrinkles?

**A** Damage occurs to the collagen and elastin fibers in the reticular dermis over time. Expression lines are caused by a gradual "denting" of these fibers from repeated facial movement. Just like a piece of metal that is bent multiple times, the fibers become weaker and thinner in the area of the constant bend.

If you carefully examine the tissue of sun-damaged skin, you will find a disorganized mess in the reticular dermis. Both collagen and elastin fibers are damaged from cumulative sun exposure. Little by little, these fibers are damaged until they cannot function in their intended capacity. This damage results in both skin wrinkling medically known as **rhytides** and skin sagging known as **elastosis.**

**Q** Is there more than one type of skin wrinkling?

**A** There are two main types of skin wrinkles: those caused by facial expressions, called **expression lines,** and those caused by cumulative sun damage. The facial expression lines are in the areas of constant repeated facial movement. These include horizontal forehead lines, "scowl" lines between the eyes, crow's-feet at the outside corners of the eyes, and **nasolabial folds** from the corners of the mouth to the nose.

Lines caused from sun exposure are medically termed **solar rhytides.** These wrinkles are not necessarily in the areas of facial movement; they are often criss-cross wrinkles and can be in any area of the face, neck, or chest.

**Q** What causes skin to sag when it gets older?

**A** If you gently pinch the skin, it should snap back quickly. Older skin and sun-damaged skin do not return to form quickly. Elastin fibers in the dermis are responsible for the ability of the skin to "snap back" and return to its original shape. As the skin ages, elastin fibers become stretched out due to facial movement and gravity constantly pulling down on the skin and the body. Cumulative sun damage also damages these fibers, resulting in elastosis, which is failure of the skin to return to its original form, ultimately resulting in sagging skin.

**Q.** **How much does heredity have to do with how someone's skin ages?**

**A** You only have to look at a mother and daughter or look through a family album to know that genetics does have an effect on facial aging. How many times have you heard "he looks just like his dad"? We inherit facial features, bone structure, muscle structure, oiliness or dryness, baldness tendencies, atopic eczema, allergies, and, to some extent, how the skin holds up over the years.

We also inherit ethnic skin characteristics, including skin coloration that can determine our natural defense against sun exposure.

In addition, we inherit skin care and health habits. If our parents do not practice good skin care or health habits, we will have a tendency not to practice them either. It is important to teach children good health habits, to use sunscreen daily, and to take good care of their skin!

**Q.** **What does skin color have to do with aging?**

**A** Skin color has a direct correlation with tendencies to facial aging and sun damage. There is a well-known measurement scale called **Fitzpatrick Skin Typing** that classifies skin coloration into six different skin color categories. Each category has a different resistance to sun exposure, tendency to burn, and tendency to sun-related aging damage. The lower the number classification, the more likely the skin is to be damaged by the sun, and the more likely it is to have premature aging appearance.

- Type I—This skin is very fair, usually with blue or green eyes, red or blonde hair, and often hereditarily freckled skin. It always burns when exposed to the sun and never tans.
- Type II—This skin burns easily and tans only minimally. Again, the skin color is fair, with blue, green, or hazel eyes, and with blonde or red hair.
- Type III—Many people have this skin coloring. Still considered fair, this skin type will gradually tan if exposed to sun but can still burn. They can have any color hair and eyes.
- Type IV—Mediterranean Caucasian skin with medium to heavy pigmentation is an exemplar of this type. It almost always tans when repeatedly exposed to sun and rarely burns.
- Type V—Middle Eastern coloring with dark hair and eyes is an example of this type. This skin type is not sun-sensitive and always tans.
- Type VI—This type is black skin that is not sun sensitive.

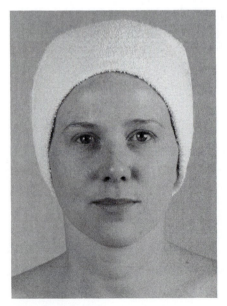

Fitzpatrick Type I.

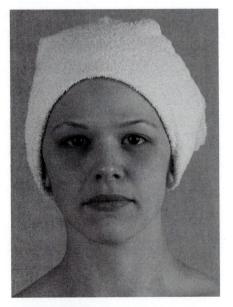

Fitzpatrick Type II.

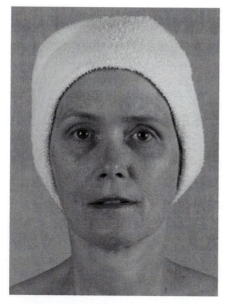

Fitzpatrick Type III.

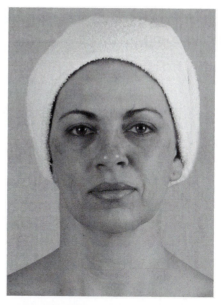

Fitzpatrick Type IV.

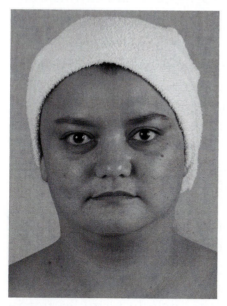

Fitzpatrick Type V.

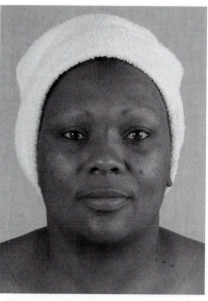

Fitzpatrick Type VI.

Darker skin types have more natural pigment protection against sun exposure. Persons with darker skin are also a lot less likely to deliberately expose themselves to sun in order to get a darker appearance of the skin.

**Q** What is the difference between extrinsic and intrinsic skin aging?

**A** **Intrinsic skin aging** refers to aging of the skin that occurs naturally. Hereditary factors, ethnicity, skin coloration, gravity's effect on the skin over time, and actual chronological age (the passing of years) determine signs of intrinsic aging.

**Extrinsic skin aging** is exposure and environmental factors that affect skin aging. What happens to the skin over a lifetime is extrinsic skin aging. Sun exposure, smoking, exposure to pollutants, and health habits that affect the skin are all factors in extrinsic skin aging. Extrinsic factors affecting the skin are generally controllable and avoidable, which makes the extrinsic signs of aging preventable!

**Q** How can you tell which aging symptoms are extrinsic and which intrinsic?

**A** Gravity's effect on the skin, which mainly involves a slow, gradual sagging of the skin over the decades, is the primary intrinsic aging characteristic. The development of expression lines from repeated facial movement is also intrinsic. Smile lines, crow's-feet around the eyes, horizontal forehead lines, and the "eleven" lines between the eyes are all intrinsic expression lines. In later years, cartilage in the nose and ears starts to grow, making the ears and nose larger.

Another intrinsic factor is a gradual thinning of the subcutaneous fat in the face in the later years. This generally begins in the 60s and is evident in a "bony" appearance of the faces of older persons.

Extrinsic aging is primarily caused by cumulative sun exposure. Signs of sun damage include wrinkles not in the facial expression, deeper facial expression lines, crisscross wrinkling, severe skin sagging, multiple discolorations and hyperpigmentation, rough or leathery textured skin, distended capillaries, and skin growths including skin cancers.

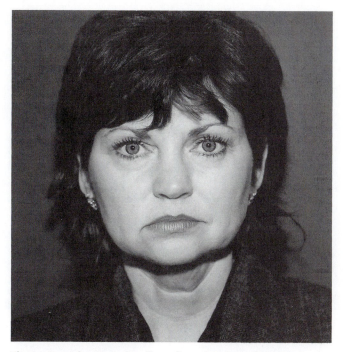

Elastosis and expression lines from intrinsic factors
*(courtesy Derek A. Jones, M.D., F.A.C.S.).*

The medical term for skin damage from sun exposure is **dermatoheliosis.** Skin that is damaged from extrinsic factors will appear much older than skin of the same age that only has intrinsic aging factors.

One of the main and first-appearing signs of dermatoheliosis is splotchy discoloration of the skin. This is caused by the skin trying to defend itself against sun exposure. A tan is actually an immune function of the skin, desperately trying to shield itself from the sun's damaging rays!

The damage caused by sun exposure is cumulative, and so are its symptoms. What appears as a golden tan in the 20s will appear as wrinkles, pigment splotchiness, and even skin cancers at age 40.

**Q** How is inflammation related to skin aging symptoms?

**A** Chronic inflammation of the skin, especially including cumulative sun exposure, causes a domino effect of

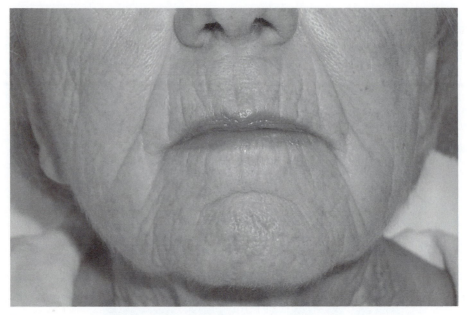

Dermatoheliosis—aging from sun damage.

biochemical reactions called the **inflammation cascade,** also known as the **free radical cascade.** Inflammation results in the formation of **free radicals,** which are unstable atoms that rob electrons from cells in the skin, that can cause damage to DNA in cells and the fibroblasts that produce collagen. Free radicals also produce biochemical damage that can lead to eventual skin cancers and abnormal growths. The end products of this inflammatory biochemical reaction can cause the skin to produce "self-destruct" enzymes such as collagenase, elastase, and hyaluronidase, which destroy collagen, elastin, and hyaluronic acid. These "little destructive insults" happen each day that your skin is exposed to the sun without protection. When enough of this damage accumulates, we see signs of wrinkles, elastosis, and other evidence of sun damage.

**Q** **What can be done to control inflammation in the skin?**

**A** First and foremost, prevention of inflammation can be achieved by the daily use of sunscreen. Avoidance of sources that cause inflammation, such as constant exposure to heat or the overuse of skin care treatments that chronically leave the skin inflamed, will prevent inflammation-related damage. Lastly, the use of both topical and internal antioxidants can help inhibit these destructive reactions before they damage the skin.

**Q** **What role do hormones play in skin aging?**

**A** A female hormone called **estrogen** is needed for production of collagen in the dermis. After menopause, the estrogen production in females is drastically reduced. This may result in less supple skin, an increase in wrinkling, and elastosis.

Hormones also play roles in pigmentation and blood circulation, which may influence hyperpigmentation and redness issues in the aging skin. Perimenopausal acne and facial hair growth may affect some women during and after menopause.

**Q** **Why does older skin have age spots?**

**A** Age spots, also sometimes called liver spots—which have nothing to do with liver, except perhaps they are of a similar

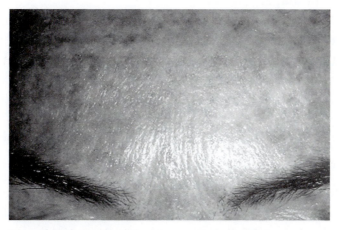

Sun-related pigmentation *(courtesy Mark Lees Skin Care, Inc.)*.

color—are signs of dermatoheliosis and cumulative sun damage. They have more to do with sun exposure than they do with age. Melanocytes, the pigment-producing cells in the skin, are overproducing melanin in these areas. The spots are known medically as **solar lentigines.** They can appear anywhere on the body but are most frequently on the face and hands, which are areas constantly exposed to the sun. We will discuss treatment for these in Chapter 7.

**Q** Is barrier function a factor in mature skin?

**A** The barrier function is a matrix of fatty components between the cells in the epidermis produced during the epidermal keratinization process. This fatty "mortar" between the "bricks" (epidermal cells) prevents transepidermal water loss from the inside out, and it prevents irritant penetration from the outside in.

As the skin gets older, the epidermal cell cycle slows down substantially. This slowing reduces the production of intercellular lipids, creating probable impaired barrier function. Impaired barrier function can result in dehydration, which makes wrinkling and skin texture much worse. Impaired barrier also allows irritants to more easily penetrate the skin. These irritants can lead to inflammation, which can cause damage.

Barrier function can be repaired with the use of lipid-infused moisturizers and serums, and skin can be protected by not using stripping cleansers and using proper protectants that can guard against barrier damage.

**Q** What can be done to help the appearance of the aging skin?

**A** There are numerous scientific treatment concepts to help improve the appearance of aging skin symptoms:

- **Use of a broad-spectrum daily sunscreen** with an SPF of at least 15 will help prevent inflammation and sun damage. Prevention is the best concept in treatment of aging skin and skin suffering from dermatoheliosis.

- **Daily use of topical antioxidants** helps inhibit inflammatory reactions that can lead to skin damage. These may include ingredients such as green tea, grape-seed extract, magnesium ascorbyl phosphate (vitamin C ester), tocopherol (vitamin E), licorice extracts, and others.
- **Protection and repair of the barrier function** restores intercellular hydration and protection. This is accomplished by using products that contain ingredients that help patch the barrier function, including glycolipids, ceramides, fatty acids, and cholesterol—the exact components of the natural barrier function. This reduces inflammation and hydrates the skin properly, improving smoothness of the skin and improving skin health in general.
- **Daily use of chemical exfoliants** such as alpha hydroxy acids helps to accelerate slowing cell renewal,

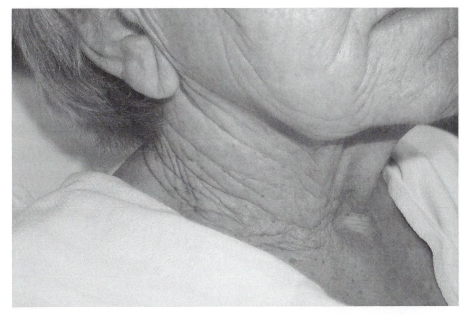

Sun-related aging is characterized by wrinkles and elastosis.

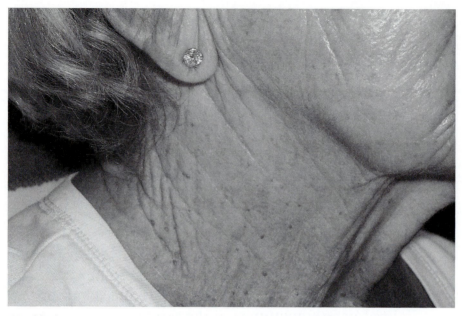

Wrinkled appearance greatly improved in 8 weeks by combining regular usage of daily sunscreen, alpha hydroxy acids, peptides, and lipids.

smooth rough surface textures, and improve the appearance of wrinkles.

- **Collagen stimulation** can be achieved through the use of alpha hydroxy acids and botanical stimulant ingredients such as plant extracts *Centella asiatica* and *Echinacea angustifolia*.

- **Peptides** are one of newest beneficial ingredient types for influencing or modulating aging skin to behave like younger skin. Peptides are being used to improve skin elasticity, reduce the appearance of expression lines, reduce puffiness, and provide other helpful changes.

- **Hydration** may be old school, but it is vitally important for skin to function well. Use of the right moisturizer on a daily basis is essential. All of the modern science will not work if the skin is dehydrated!

**Q** What should I look for in a good sunscreen product for me?

**A** Besides avoidance of sun exposure, daily use of sunscreen is the most important preventive technique to avoid premature aging of the skin. There are several things you should look for in a sunscreen:

- Make sure that the sunscreen is **broad-spectrum,** which means that it screens both UVA and UVB rays. This generally means that it will have a mix of active ingredients on the label.
- The sunscreen should have an SPF of at least 15.
- The last factor is very important. Most importantly: You must find a sunscreen product that you really like and can comfortably use every day, and that can double as a moisturizer. It is important that it is easily workable into your skin care regimen. Wearing a moisturizer with built-in sunscreen is an easy health habit that can make a world of difference to any skin.

Moisturizers with built-in sunscreen protection are available in many different weights and now designed for many skin types, including oily, combination, dry, or sensitive skin.

For more detailed information on sunscreens, see Chapter 6.

**Q** **Is it important that the sunscreen is water-resistant?**

**A** You only need a water-resistant sunscreen if you work outside, expect to perspire heavily, or know you will be wet during the day. Most people who have normal indoor jobs do not need a water resistant sunscreen for daily activities. Water-resistant sunscreens tend to be heavy and not suitable for pre-makeup use.

A water-resistant sunscreen is necessary for swimming, beach activity, outdoor sports, and prolonged outdoor activity.

**Q** **Why is UVA and UVB broad-spectrum protection important?**

**A** The two main rays from the sun are **ultraviolet alpha (UVA)** and **ultraviolet beta (UVB).** UVB rays are shorter rays that cause sunburns and most common skin cancers. UVA rays are much longer and deeper-penetrating, and are believed to cause the most damage in terms of premature skin aging, elastosis, and wrinkling. They are both implicated in skin cancer formation, including melanoma.

**Q** **What can be done to improve the barrier function of aging skin?**

**A** As previously discussed, the barrier function in older skin is affected by both the intrinsic slowing of the cell renewal cycle and cumulative extrinsic damage from sun and inflammation. Additionally, many people with mature skin produce less protective sebum, making barrier function damage even more likely.

Impaired barrier function can result in dry, flaky, dehydrated skin as well as redness and inflammation. Impaired barrier function can also result in a "deflated" look to the skin surface, making wrinkles and elastosis look worse.

Restored barrier function can make a tremendous difference in the smoothness, suppleness, and hydration of the skin. Skin with a good barrier function is firmer looking and is much less likely to show signs of inflammation or redness.

Barrier function can be restored or improved by the following:

- Using gentle cleansers prevents overstripping of the protective barrier on the surface of the skin. Over-cleansing or cleansing too frequently can strip the protective sebum layer and begin affecting the barrier lipids between the epidermal cells. Choose cleansers that do not foam or foam lightly, which indicates a low level of detergent content. A cleanser designed for sensitive skin and tested for irritancy would be a good choice for most dry aging skin types. Toners should be free of drying alcohols.

■ Use products that are infused with lipids. It is possible to "patch" the barrier function by using products that contain complexes that mimic or substitute for the natural barrier lipids. These products will contain a complex of sphingolipids, phospholipids, fatty acids, and cholesterol, which together comprise the natural barrier function lipid matrix. This complex can be used in moisturizers, sunscreens, eye creams, masks, or intensive serums. Lipid-infused products are excellent choices for dry skin in general.

■ Use alpha hydroxy acids to help restore a normal cell renewal cycle. It is the normal keratinization process that produces the natural barrier lipids. Alpha hydroxy acids (AHAs) work to remove dead, dry surface cells, stimulating their replacement and the production of barrier lipids. Studies have shown significant barrier repair resulting from the use of AHAs.

**Q** What are the benefits of using topical antioxidants?

**A** Antioxidants work by neutralizing free radicals, interrupting the inflammation cascade. They do this by binding or furnishing electrons to the electron-starved free radicals.

Antioxidants, therefore, stop free radicals from causing damage to the cells. This cannot be immediately seen visually. The protection of the skin by antioxidants has wonderful long-term effects, helping the skin stay healthy and younger looking. You can look at the use of antioxidants as you might look at taking a daily multivitamin. You don't usually see immediate results taking vitamins, but long-range you are helping your body stay healthy. Some of the vitamins we take are also antioxidants!

Some antioxidants do have a strong soothing, anti-inflammatory effect on reddened skin. Green tea, lichochalcone (licorice extract), and grapeseed extract are examples of redness-quenching antioxidants.

**Q** **What are some popular antioxidant ingredients and which are the best?**

**A** Vitamin C (l-ascorbic acid or magnesium ascorbyl phosphate), vitamin E (tocopherol or tocopheryl acetate), grapeseed extract, lichochalcone or stearyl glycyrrhetinate (extracts from licorice), green tea extract, superoxide dismutase, and coenzyme Q-10 are all examples of popular antioxidants. Other ingredients also have antioxidant activity.

There are many types of free radicals in the inflammation cascade and numerous biochemical reactions that create new types of free radicals. Whenever a free radical steals electrons from another atom, this creates another free radical, but it may be different from the original free radical.

For example, most free radicals begin as simple oxygen. Oxygen is the original source of most free radicals because it is extremely reactive and, when in an excited state, needs electrons to stabilize it. Free radical oxygen may steal electrons from a skin cell membrane. When this happens, the oxygen is stabilized, but the lipids attacked in the cell membrane are now missing electrons and have become a different type of free radical called **lipid peroxide,** which now can react with another atom and create another different radical.

Because of the many types of radicals that can be formed in the cascade of reactions, more than one type of antioxidant is needed to squelch these reactions. Different antioxidants work in different ways on different radicals. Therefore, a mix of antioxidants is the best bet in helping the aging skin.

**Q** **What should I look for in an antioxidant product?**

**A** Antioxidants are reactive and must be carefully formulated so that they do not oxidize. Oxidized antioxidants are antioxidants that have been used and are no longer effective. One of the signs of an oxidized product is that it begins turning dark and eventually turns brown in the bottle.

Good antioxidant products are formulated to protect the antioxidant so it will work on the skin instead of in the bottle. Often, liposomes are used to protect the ingredients in the product. Antioxidant products should be stored in a cool place and not exposed to constant light.

Serums are one of the most popular forms of antioxidants because they can be easily layered under another product. Antioxidant serums are most often applied after cleansing and toning the skin and before other treatment products, moisturizer, or sunscreen.

**Q** What effect does daily chemical exfoliation have on aging skin?

**A** **Chemical exfoliation** is the use of a product that dissolves or loosens dead cell buildup. **Mechanical exfoliation** removes surface cells by physically bumping them off the skin. A scrub is an example of a mechanical exfoliator.

Using a daily chemical exfoliant such as alpha hydroxy acid can make a huge difference in skin that already has aging symptoms, and it can actually help maintain younger-looking skin. Mechanical exfoliators are good for helping make the skin look smoother and clearer but do not have the same long-range effects as daily-use chemical exfoliants.

**Alpha hydroxy acids (AHAs)** include glycolic, lactic, mandelic, malic, and tartaric acids. The most popular of this group are glycolic and lactic acids. **Beta hydroxy acids (BHAs)** include salicylic and citric acids. Salicylic acid is also used as a chemical exfoliant and is sometimes used in conjunction with AHAs.

By loosening and removing dead surface cells, chemical exfoliants accomplish the following:

- Removal of dead cell buildup on the skin's surface immediately causes a smoothing effect on the skin, reflecting light more evenly and making wrinkles look less deep.

- Small epidermal lines are significantly lessened, often to the point where they are no longer visible. Continual use produces continued improvement in skin smoothness.
- Daily use of AHAs speeds up the epidermal cell renewal, significantly improving hydration, helping to plump the skin surface cells, and improving smoothness and texture.
- With daily use of AHAs, the barrier function is improved due to the acceleration of the cell renewal cycle.

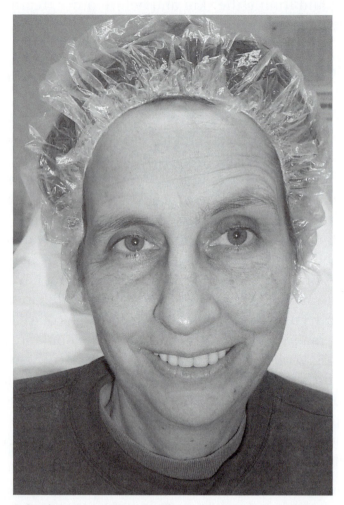

Splotchy, uneven pigmentation is typical of sun-related aging even in younger clients.

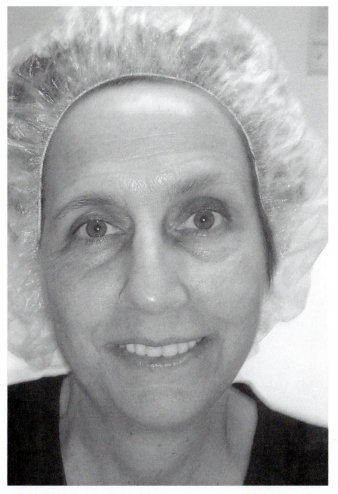

Regular use of an alpha hydroxy serum, peptides, antioxidants, and sunscreen can make a huge difference in the reduction of signs of aging.

- Routine use of daily AHAs stimulates the production of new collagen in the skin, adding to skin firmness.
- Daily chemical exfoliation removes stained or hyper-pigmented dead cells, improving the appearance of dark spots, sun-related freckles, and splotchiness. Chemical exfoliants are also often combined with lightening or brightening products to help increase penetration of the lightening agents.

**Q** How do I know which type of alpha hydroxy home-care product is right for my skin?

**A** Alpha hydroxy acid products are available in cream, lotion, serum, and gel forms. They are worn on the skin, usually under a moisturizer or sunscreen. You should choose the product that is most appropriate for your skin type. Creams are most often intended for drier skin, and gels are best for oily and combination skin. Serums can often be used on several skin types. If you are not sure, ask your skin care professional to help you choose the right product for your skin.

The percentage of alpha hydroxy acid content is important. Make sure the product contains 8–10% alpha hydroxy acid. Some products are blends of more than one AHA. It is the total percentage that is important. Products with more than 10% AHA can cause inflammation and visible peeling of the skin, which is not necessary in order to see results with an AHA product.

Another important factor is the pH of the product, which, simply put, measures the acidic value of the product. Ideally, an AHA product should have a pH of about 3.5 and an AHA concentration of 8–10%. Products with pHs lower than 3.5, when used on a daily basis, can cause inflammation and irritation.

Some cleansers and scrubs contain AHAs. Rinse-off products do not produce the same improvement effects on the skin as a product that is worn.

Sunscreen use is imperative when using alpha hydroxy acid products. Because the surface is being routinely exfoliated, the skin must be protected from UV exposure.

**Q** What are peptides and how do they help the skin?

**A** **Peptides** are chains of amino acids. Chains of peptides form proteins. There are many different types of peptides because there are many types of amino acids, and many combinations can be formed.

The entire body, including the skin, is run by biochemical reactions. Peptides are thought to send signals or somehow stimulate the skin to behave in a different way. It is believed that certain sequences of amino acids produce different effects when exposed to the skin.

The first, and probably the most well-known in skin care products, peptide is called **palmitoyl pentapeptide-3,** commercially known as Matrixyl. This peptide helps to improve the firmness of the skin. Research has documented that this peptide stimulates collagen production in the skin and also increases the amount of water-binding substances in the dermis. Regular use of a properly formulated product containing palmitoyl pentapeptide-3 can improve the appearance of fine lines, wrinkles, firmness, and elasticity. The ingredient has no known side effects and there have been no reports of irritation.

Another well-known, and popular due to advertising its attributes peptide is **acetyl hexapeptide-3,** commercially known as Argireline. Acetyl hexapeptide-3 has anti-wrinkle properties and is often promoted and used to treat expression lines, but it can be used on any type of wrinkle. The peptide works by inhibiting certain binding proteins that create the tension that causes wrinkling.

There are other types of peptides now available in skin care products that can help with elasticity, puffiness, fluid retention, and other esthetic problems. There will likely be many new peptide ingredients available in the future, since we have just recently discovered this way to change the skin's behavior to improve the skin appearance.

Peptides are being used in serums, moisturizers, eye creams, and other types of products. To have a real lasting effect on the skin, peptide products must be used consistently, and solid results cannot be expected from periodic use.

Peptides can be used in conjunction with other products to minimize the appearance of aging, including sunscreens, AHA products, antioxidants, lipid-based products, and moisturizers. A combination of all of these ingredient types in a planned program for daily application can produce substantial improvement in the appearance of age- or sun damage–related wrinkling, elastosis, puffiness, and other visible signs of age or dermatoheliosis.

**Q** **What are the different types of peels?**

**A** There are several levels of peels:

- **Deep peels,** also sometimes called *surgical peels,* should be performed only by dermatologists and plastic surgeons and remove the entire epidermis and dermal tissue. This peel requires sedation or anesthesia and also requires pain medication during recovery. This deep peel, usually performed with phenol, is performed to treat severe sun damage and very deep and widespread wrinkling. It takes up to 6–8 weeks to heal and can take several additional months before the redness from the peel subsides.
- **Medium depth peels** are performed using trichloroacetic acid (TCA). This peel removes the entire epidermis and also removes some dermal tissue. Again, only a dermatologist or plastic surgeon should perform this peel. Some estheticians use a lower strength TCA peel, but it is this author's opinion that TCA should be reserved for qualified physician's hands.
- **Superficial peels** are light peels that only remove corneum cells from the epidermis. They utilize mild acids or enzymes to remove or dissolve the surface keratinocytes. They are performed by licensed estheticians and may also be performed in dermatology or plastic surgery clinics. Superficial peels do not peel beyond the surface cells and do not cause any blistering or bleeding. Some may produce temporary discomfort, but, in general, they do not cause any great pain. They require no major recovery time, and most people have no visible side effects.

**Q** How can peels help the aging skin?

**A** Superficial peels performed by licensed estheticians work by removing a portion of the corneum, the outside layer of the epidermis. Like peeling the outside of an onion, superficial peels can make the skin look a lot smoother, helping to improve rough textures and reducing the depth of surface lines and wrinkles. It is especially effective in improving the look of surface "crepiness" and fine lines around the eyes.

Superficial peels also remove dead pigmented cells, fading splotchiness and improving solar-induced hyperpigmentation.

The most common type of superficial peel administered by estheticians is the alpha hydroxy acid (AHA) peel. Sometimes called exfoliation treatments, these AHA treatments are about three times the concentration of a home care AHA treatment product and have a slightly lower pH, usually around 3.0. They are generally performed in a series of six, usually administered once or twice a week, depending on the peel product and the condition and sensitivity of the skin to be treated. The skin must be prepared for this peel treatment by using an 8–10% AHA homecare product on a daily basis for at least 2 weeks before the series of treatments begins. Sunscreen must also be worn on a daily basis. It is best to plan such a series at a time when you are not planning to have extensive outdoor exposure for the next few weeks. AHA treatment series can be performed safely 2–3 times a year, and maintenance AHA treatments are also available, usually once or twice a month, depending on the strength and pH of the particular peel product used.

Salicylic acid peels are also sometimes used by estheticians. These are slightly stronger than most AHA peels and are administered less often.

Jessner's peels are a chemical combination of salicylic acid, resorcinol, and lactic acid. They are the strongest peels estheticians usually use without medical supervision. The strength of this peel varies with the number of application coats of the liquid peel. Jessner's peels are frequently used to treat hyperpigmentation as well as wrinkles and texture problems.

Jessner's peels cause visible peeling and flaking of the skin for several days after the application. The amount of peeling depends on the number of layers of peel product applied. Anyone planning to have a Jessner's treatment should make sure that they aware of the number of recovery days required because of the skin peeling factor.

**Q** **Does oily skin age differently than dry skin?**

**A** Oily skin often seems to age less than dry skin, but it is probably because oily skin tends to be thicker hereditarily than dry skin types. Thicker skin, however, has a tendency to form more pronounced and deeper looking expression lines.

Darker skin types tend to be oilier and also have more protective pigment that serves as natural protection against the sun.

Oily skin does have more of a protective layer of sebum than dry skin, and it is less likely to suffer from dehydration or barrier function damage that can make wrinkles and rough skin texture look worse.

Sun damage, however, can occur in either skin type, and wrinkling, elastosis, and other sun-related problems can affect both oily and dry skin.

**Q** **What can be done about around-the-mouth wrinkles?**

**A** Those pesky wrinkles, known as **perioral rhytides,** are much more likely to happen to women than men. Sometimes called "smoker's lines," these vertical lines across the top and bottom of the lips can also occur when someone is not a smoker. Mouth lines on a smoker, however, are more likely to be deeper and occur sooner.

It is repeated expressions that cause these lines to form. They rarely occur in men, mainly due to a structural difference in the skin and muscle fibers surrounding the mouth area. Skin care treatments to help soften these lines include home-care use of alpha hydroxy acid serum or cream, regular application of an acetyl hexapeptide product, and use of lipids to improve hydration.

AHAs will help to reduce the wrinkle depth from the skin surface. Acetyl hexapeptide will help to loosen the tension of the wrinkles, and lipids will help to boost moisture levels to plump out the epidermis.

The lines can also be treated by a plastic surgeon or dermatologist with filler injections, such as Restylane (hyaluronic acid), or they can be treated by laser. Lines around the mouth can be difficult to treat, and even after medical treatment, they sometimes reoccur.

**Q** **Is micro-current helpful for aging skin?**

**A** **Micro-current** is a gentle electrical current applied to the skin with probes. Micro-current is used by estheticians to stimulate the skin, and it can be used to help many different skin problems.

Micro-current use in aging skin focuses on the muscle structure of the face. The facial skin is attached to the muscles of the face. Nowhere else on the body is muscle attachment the same as on the face.

As skin feels the effect of gravity over the years, the muscles also feel this effect, and they are not as tight or toned as they were earlier in life.

Micro-current can be used to "re-train" the facial muscles, resulting in a tightened structure. When the muscle is tightened, the skin is lifted by the improved muscle structure. These treatments, often referred to as "liftings" or "tonings" by estheticians, can be helpful in skin with poor elasticity. They also can be alternated with other treatments such as AHA peels and LED light therapy for a multitherapy approach.

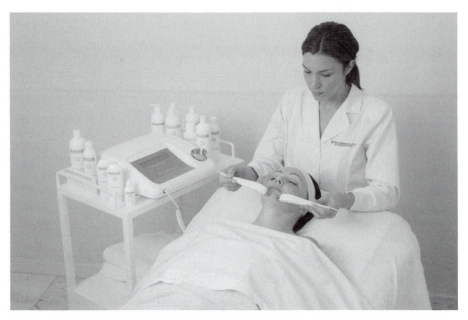

Micro-current treatments are used to improve skin tone and elasticity *(courtesy Bio-Therapeutic, Inc.)*.

Micro-current has also been documented to increase the elastin content of the skin and increase the ATP (adenosine triphosphate) in the cells. ATP is the main source of energy for cells to function properly.

**Q** **How often are the micro-current treatments performed?**

**A** Micro-current must be administered in a series of treatments, usually beginning with two or three treatments per week for 12 treatments. Skin that is severely sun damaged may require a longer introductory series. The results must be maintained with treatments at least once or twice a month. If the treatments are discontinued, the muscle and skin will both return to their original condition.

Think of micro-current as you would think of working out at a gym. To get your body in shape, you must have frequent workouts and be disciplined until you have achieved the results you want. Then, you must continue the workouts, even if not as frequently, to maintain your body's new look.

**Q.** **Does micro-current therapy change the need for home care?**

**A** Absolutely not! Home care is essential for good skin. Micro-current treatment will enhance and boost your home-care results.

**Q.** **How does light therapy affect the skin?**

**A** Estheticians use **light-emitting diodes (LED)** equipment to treat the appearance of the signs of aging. These intense flashing light rays are flashing so fast that they cannot be seen by the human eye. Exposing the skin to this flashing light stimulates production of collagen in the skin and can also be used to treat redness, acne, and other conditions.

LED therapy needs to be administered in a series of treatments to be most effective and have long-lasting results. Maintenance treatments are also recommended.

**Intense pulsed light (IPL)** is a more invasive form of light therapy used by physicians to treat distended capillaries, treat hyperpigmentation, and perform hair reduction.

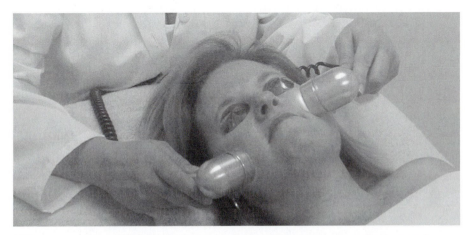

LED treatments use flashing lights to improve the appearance of aging and redness *(courtesy Revitalight)*.

**Q** Is facial exercise helpful for aging skin?

**A** You would think so, considering what we just discussed how muscles in the face are connected to the skin. Facial muscles will tighten with exercise, but it is hard to isolate facial muscles, making it difficult to change the structure. The main problem with facial exercise is that it also causes pronounced facial expressions and can make expression lines worse.

Micro-current can be applied to isolated muscles and does not cause visible muscle contraction, so it does not cause facial expression. Some muscles, like the ones around the mouth, need to be relaxed and elongated instead of contracted. This also can be accomplished with micro-current, but not with exercise.

**Q** What can be done about smile lines and worry lines?

**A** Esthetic treatment involves treatment of these areas at home with alpha hydroxy acid and acetyl hexapeptide as previously discussed for lines around the mouth. Micro-current can also help soften these lines.

Medically, a plastic surgeon or dermatologist can inject the muscle with Botox (botulinum toxin), which will temporarily paralyze the muscle to stop the facial expressions that cause the frown lines.

Botox is usually not used in the mouth area. Smile lines can be injected with a filler such as Restylane. The filler "plumps" the tissue inside the wrinkle, making it less deep and less visible.

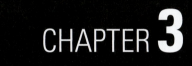

# CHAPTER 3

# Acne and
# Acne-Prone Skin

**Q** **Why do pores develop?**

**A** A pore is a lay term usually referring to the appearance of the openings of the follicles on the skin's surface. When someone complains about having large pores, they are complaining about the visible size of their follicle openings.

Consumers often use the terms *pore* and *follicle* interchangeably when discussing clogged pores, which are actually follicles clogged with dead cell buildup and solidified sebum. The follicle is a duct in the skin that contains a hair and is attached to the sebaceous glands that produce sebum. It is from the bottom of a follicle that a hair grows and through a follicle that sebum finds its way to the skin surface to lubricate the surface.

If you look at the skin of an infant or toddler, you may comment about the beautiful "peaches and cream" complexion, appearing completely pore-less. However, at this point in life, the follicles are there, collapsed and invisible to the naked eye. They do not become obvious until

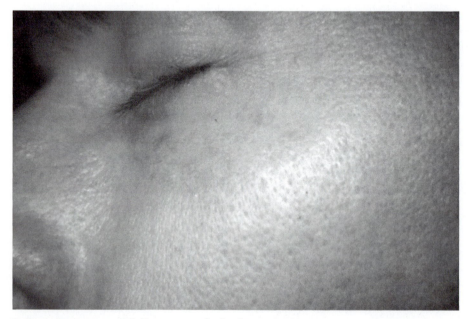

Enlarged pores are a definite sign of oily skin.

sebum begins being produced by the sebaceous glands, around the age of puberty. The sebum flow through the follicle stretches the follicle walls, creating the visible opening called *pores* by consumers. You can think of it as a collapsed garden hose that appears to be flat until someone connects the hose to a faucet and turns on the water. At that point the hose fills out to allow water to flow through it.

**Q** What role does heredity play in oily and acne-prone skin?

**A** Heredity is a key factor in acne-prone and oily skin. There are several important characteristics that are hereditary and passed on genetically from parent to child. Oily skin and oiliness levels are hereditary. The number, size, and productivity of the sebaceous glands is determined by genetics. Hormones can influence oiliness levels, but even hormonal activity is influenced by hereditary factors.

People who have oily skin often complain about the size of their pores, how they cannot keep makeup on their faces due to the oiliness, and always ask what can be done. The truth is that even though there are many things that can be done to control oiliness, it cannot be permanently corrected because oiliness is hereditary.

Acne-prone skin and oily skin types do not shed cells from the skin surface or from the lining of the follicle in the same way that normal skin does. **Retention hyperkeratosis** is a technical term for the hereditary tendency of this skin type to not shed cells, and therefore have "pile-ups" of dead cells. Hyperkeratosis means "cell buildup." The cells build up inside the follicles, thickening the lining of the follicle and contributing to the congestion of the follicles, resulting in the formation of clogged pores, blackheads, and other impactions.

Sebum coats the buildup of cells on the follicle walls. Sebum also tends to oxidize and harden into a solidified mass of dead cells and hardened sebum. This mass is difficult, if not impossible, for the skin follicle to expel.

The tendency to the formation of cysts and scar tissue is also genetic. Persons who have grade 4 (cystic) acne carry genes for the development of this severe and possibly disfiguring skin condition. Scarring can occur in individual acne lesions in many people with acne; however, the strong tendency toward severe scarring is hereditary.

**Q** **What causes blackheads?**

**A** The previously discussed hereditary oiliness problem and retention hyperkeratosis are major contributors to the formation of **open comedones**. Open comedones are also known as blackheads and occur in oily skin areas.

These unattractive dilated follicles are caused by a buildup of dead cells in the follicle and the mixture of this buildup with the sebum secreted by the sebaceous glands. The sebum solidifies in the follicles, forming a hardened mass of fatty materials mixed with dead cells from the hyperkeratosis.

Many people erroneously think that the black part of a blackhead is dirt. The darkening of the sebum on the tip of an open comedo is actually caused by oxidation. The follicle is dilated to the point where the sebum oxidizes, forming a dark "head" on the surface of the sebum impactions from exposure to the air.

Blackheads rarely develop into any other form of acne lesion. Because of the dilated follicle in an open comedo, oxygen can easily penetrate the sides and lower levels of the follicle. This oxygen kills off acne bacteria, *Propionibacterium acnes*, which are anaerobic bacteria. Anaerobic bacteria cannot survive in the presence of oxygen. To summarize, no one likes having open comedones (blackheads), but they rarely develop into inflammatory acne lesions such as papules and pustules. Because they do not change and there is no break in the follicle wall, open comedones are referred to as noninflammatory lesions.

**Q** **Are the tiny clogged pores I get on my nose the same as open comedones?**

**A** No. These tiny clogged follicles are called **sebaceous filaments.** Sebaceous filaments are similar to open comedones, but they are obviously much smaller and they contain mostly solidified, hardened sebum and little cell buildup. The black head of the lesion is caused by oxidation of the sebum exposed to the atmosphere at the top of the follicle.

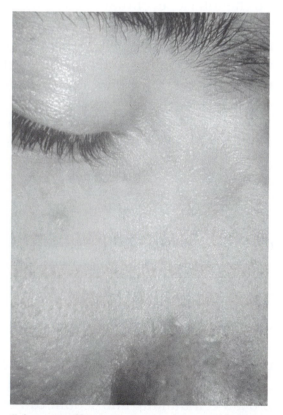

Sebaceous filaments, as seen here in the corner of the nose, are follicles filled with oxidized sebum. They are found in very oily areas of the face *(courtesy Mark Lees Skin Care, Inc.)*.

**Q** How does a pimple form?

**A** As previously discussed, retention hyperkeratosis and oiliness from hereditarily active sebaceous glands causes a buildup of dead cells in skin follicles that are bound together by sticky and solidified sebum. These dead cells begin clumping together in the bottom of skin follicles. This clumping is known as a **microcomedo**. Microcomedones are the beginning of all acne lesions. They cannot be seen with the naked eye. Because they cannot be seen, they are often ignored and not treated. The real trick to controlling all forms of acne is treating and preventing the formation of microcomedones!

From this "clumping" stage, more dead cell buildup and sebum contribute to the follicle, eventually filling with this "clumpy" debris.

If the follicle and follicle opening, the **ostium,** dilate during the pileup of clumping, the sebum on the surface oxidizes and therefore darkens, forming the previously discussed open comedo or blackhead.

If the follicle does not dilate, the buildup occurs in the follicle and cannot oxidize due to the tiny follicle opening. Congested follicles with tiny follicle openings are called **closed comedones.**

All skin follicles contain acne bacteria (*Propionibacterium acnes* or *P. acnes*). They are part of the normal bacteria that occur in the skin. *P. acnes* bacteria are **anaerobic,** which means that they only survive in the *absence* of oxygen. These bacteria, present in the bottom of the follicle, are constantly dividing (making new bacteria) *but* they are also constantly being killed by oxygen that is in the follicle.

When oxygen is blocked from the follicle, *P. acnes* bacteria can flourish and cause inflammation in the follicle. The "clumping" of dead cell buildup and sebum can block oxygen and air penetrating the follicle, allowing for the infection of the follicle. *P. acnes* bacteria break the sebum down into simpler fatty acids, which are the primary nutrition source for these bacteria.

So, in follicles congested with dead cells and solidified sebum, and if there is little or no oxygen penetrating the follicle due to the blockage or due to a small follicle opening, such as that of the closed comedo, this is an ideal environment for *P. acnes* infection.

The acne bacteria multiply and continue breaking down the sebum into fatty acids for their nourishment. In a short time, the follicle becomes swollen with bacteria, dead cells, solidified sebum, and inflammation. The follicle fills so full that the wall of the follicle ruptures or bursts. This occurs deep in the skin in the layer called the reticular dermis. As we have discussed in the questions regarding

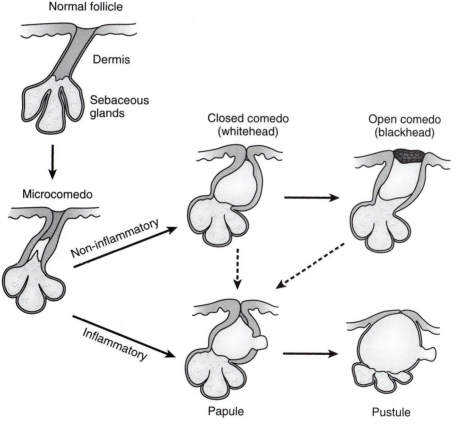

How acne lesions develop.

skin anatomy, the reticular dermis contains the blood vessels present in the skin.

The blood contains many cells that comprise the immune system. When the follicle wall breaks, a biochemical alarm alerts the immune cells within the blood that this rupture has occurred. The blood rushes to the follicle, flooding the follicle, and the white blood cells (the immune cells) within the blood begin fighting off the acne bacteria. The pimple turns red when the blood floods the follicle. At this point the lesion is called a **papule.**

During the follicle "rescue," many white blood cells, as well as acne bacteria, are killed. The dead white blood cells pile up in the follicle, along with fluids and other debris, and form a **pustule,** which is easily recognized by the white head on this pimple. Most of the pus is dead white blood cells.

**Q** Can skin care products cause or worsen acne or clogged pores?

**A** Yes, depending on the type of product. Spreading agents used in both skin care products and color cosmetics can contain fatty materials that can penetrate the follicle from the skin surface and contribute to the development of different impactions. These fatty materials may be similar to the fats in sebum that are broken down by acne bacteria in the follicles.

The tendency of a topical agent or product to cause clogged pores and comedones to develop is called **comedogenicity.** Products that cause clogging are called **comedogenic.**

Carefully check product labels to make sure they have been tested for comedogenicity. It is especially important to check products that you wear for long periods of time over acne-prone areas. This includes moisturizers and creams of all types, sunscreens, serums, foundations, powders, and blushes. Also check tanning products, bronzers, and self-tanning products to make sure they do not contain comedogenic ingredients.

**Q** What are some ingredients that are comedogenic?

**A** Most ingredients that are comedogenic are part of the **vehicle** or spreading agent in a product. Because the spreading agent is the largest part of the product, these ingredients are often used in large concentrations in the product.

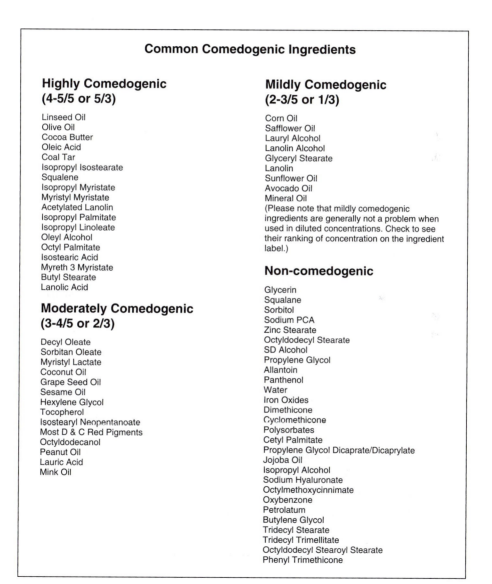

### Common Comedogenic Ingredients

**Highly Comedogenic (4-5/5 or 5/3)**

Linseed Oil
Olive Oil
Cocoa Butter
Oleic Acid
Coal Tar
Isopropyl Isostearate
Squalene
Isopropyl Myristate
Myristyl Myristate
Acetylated Lanolin
Isopropyl Palmitate
Isopropyl Linoleate
Oleyl Alcohol
Octyl Palmitate
Isostearic Acid
Myreth 3 Myristate
Butyl Stearate
Lanolic Acid

**Moderately Comedogenic (3-4/5 or 2/3)**

Decyl Oleate
Sorbitan Oleate
Myristyl Lactate
Coconut Oil
Grape Seed Oil
Sesame Oil
Hexylene Glycol
Tocopherol
Isostearyl Neopentanoate
Most D & C Red Pigments
Octyldodecanol
Peanut Oil
Lauric Acid
Mink Oil

**Mildly Comedogenic (2-3/5 or 1/3)**

Corn Oil
Safflower Oil
Lauryl Alcohol
Lanolin Alcohol
Glyceryl Stearate
Lanolin
Sunflower Oil
Avocado Oil
Mineral Oil
(Please note that mildly comedogenic ingredients are generally not a problem when used in diluted concentrations. Check to see their ranking of concentration on the ingredient label.)

**Non-comedogenic**

Glycerin
Squalane
Sorbitol
Sodium PCA
Zinc Stearate
Octyldodecyl Stearate
SD Alcohol
Propylene Glycol
Allantoin
Panthenol
Water
Iron Oxides
Dimethicone
Cyclomethicone
Polysorbates
Cetyl Palmitate
Propylene Glycol Dicaprate/Dicaprylate
Jojoba Oil
Isopropyl Alcohol
Sodium Hyaluronate
Octylmethoxycinnimate
Oxybenzone
Petrolatum
Butylene Glycol
Tridecyl Stearate
Tridecyl Trimellitate
Octyldodecyl Stearoyl Stearate
Phenyl Trimethicone

Chart of common comedogenic ingredients.

Comedogenic ingredients are often derivatives of natural oils or fatty acids, chemically altered to feel better, or lighter, on the skin or improve spreadability. Some commonly used ingredients that can be comedogenic include esters of fatty acids such as isopropyl myristate, isopropyl palmitate, decyl oleate, and myristyl myristate. Cocoa butter and coconut oil are also comedogenic. Many of the D & C red dyes, used in foundations, powders, and blushes, are also clogging. For much more information see *Skin Care: Beyond the Basics* (2007).

**Q** **Why would a company use a comedogenic ingredient in a product?**

**A** Some of the oils or fats may be helpful for skin that does not produce enough sebum. This dry skin type, however, does not have a problem with hereditary retention hyperkeratosis, and does not develop clogged pores or acne.

To have a comedogenic reaction, you must have a comedogenic product and a skin that is hereditarily acne-prone. Companies should not produce comedogenic products intended for use on oily, clog-prone, or acne-prone skin.

**Q** **What causes overnight zits?**

**A** Most of us have tried a new product and the next day had two or three pimples. Perhaps you have had pimples erupt a day or two after a facial. These reactions are called **acnegenic** reactions. Acnegenic reactions are caused by inflammation in the follicle, rather than the cell buildup and oiliness responsible for comedogenic reactions.

Acnegenic reactions may be caused by a product or action such as a facial massage, extraction, or waxing. The product or action causes inflammation of the follicle wall. If the follicle walls swell enough, they can swell into each other and obstruct the flow of oxygen in the follicle. If the oxygen is cut off, an anaerobic pocket is formed, creating an ideal environment for acne bacteria to flourish. This causes sudden "overnight" pimples.

**Q** Is there anything to look for on a product label to make sure the product is non-comedogenic and non-acnegenic?

**A** Always check the label to make sure it is safe for acne-prone or oily skin. There are laboratory tests to determine if a product is comedogenic or acnegenic. An outside independent laboratory should perform these tests. Most companies that have this testing done on their products are proud of it and will print this fact on their labels.

If you ever use a product and your skin seems to develop more clogged pores or acne lesions, stop using that product immediately.

**Q** How do you avoid acnegenic reactions?

**A** When you try a new product, make sure it is intended for acne-prone skin and that it has been tested as discussed. If you are not sure, try some in a localized area such as your forehead for a few nights before using it all over your face.

If you have acne-prone skin, you will be more likely to be sensitive to follicle-irritating products. Fragrances, essential oils, and natural oil spreading agents have all been known to cause inflammation.

**Q** I have a lot of little bumps under the skin. What are these?

**A** These tiny bumps that appear on the facial skin are likely to be small closed comedones, associated with acne. If the tiny bumps are not accompanied by other types of acne lesions, they are likely caused by comedogenic topical treatment or cosmetics.

Often, these tiny bumps appear around the hairline and on the forehead. This is known as **pomade acne.** Occlusive or comedogenic hair products, specifically hair

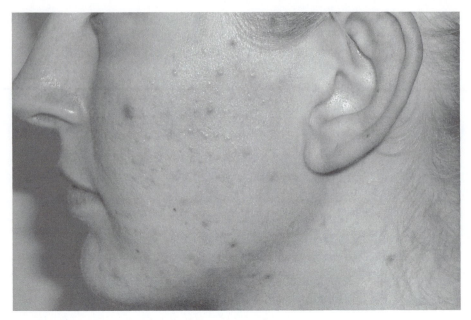

Small bumps under the skin are closed comedones *(courtesy Mark Lees Skin Care, Inc.)*.

waxes, scalp oils, some gels, some hairsprays, and other styling products, cause pomade acne. The products accidentally are applied to or migrate across the skin. This creates an occlusion on the skin surface or within the follicle.

**Q** **What can be done to help clear these hair product–related bumps?**

**A** Find a hair product that has been tested and shown to be non-comedogenic. In some cases, a tested, non-clogging facial moisturizer may be used on the hair instead of a clogging hair wax.

In general, stay away from wax type products, excessively stiff and sticky products, and anything with an oily texture. Instead, choose a water-based, non-sticky gel that dries quickly. You may want to ask your hair stylist if he or she knows of a product that will work for you without causing these bumps. Be careful not to smear product on the skin while applying it to your hair.

The daily use of both physical and chemical exfoliants will help. Use an alpha hydroxy or mild benzoyl peroxide gel in these areas lightly at night. Using a fine granular wash may help loosen surface debris and buildup causing the bumps.

**Q** **What are the basic treatment concepts for treating acne topically?**

**A** There are several basic principles for topical acne therapy:

- **Follicle exfoliation**—Daily use of a follicle exfoliant helps to gradually break up existing impactions and then prevent reoccurrence of the cell buildup that leads to impactions and formation of microcomedones. Removal of these impactions allows oxygen from the atmosphere to penetrate the follicle and kill the acne bacteria. Daily use of this product, even after the skin is clear, will help to prevent microcomedones from re-forming. Microcomedones are the initial stage of all acne lesions.

  Examples of follicle–exfoliating ingredients include benzoyl peroxide; alpha hydroxy acids such as glycolic, lactic, or mandelic acids; beta hydroxy acid; salicylic acid; sulfur; or sulfur with resorcinol. These are most often gel-based formulations.

- **Antibacterial therapy**—Benzoyl peroxide, salicylic acid, sulfur, or sulfur with resorcinol are all FDA-approved active drug ingredients for topical acne treatment. These ingredients not only help to shed the cell buildup within the follicle but also kill *P. acnes* bacteria.

- **Oil control**—Control excessive sebum by using foaming cleansers that help to break down and reduce oiliness. Choose a rinse-off wash with a cleansing agent such as ammonium lauryl sulfate. This gentle ingredient helps to remove excess oils from the skin. Some people have experienced follicle irritation using *sodium* lauryl sulfate and therefore it is not recommended for this skin type.

- Active drug ingredients such as 2½% benzoyl peroxide or salicylic acid are sometimes added to cleansers for acne skin. These may improve the cleansing product, but this is not the same as using a benzoyl peroxide or salicylic acid gel that is worn on the face overnight. Using a gel that is worn for several hours is much more effective against acne than using a rinse-off wash product.

- **Use non-comedogenic skin care**—There are some fatty-based ingredients that can cause comedones or worsen acne. These ingredients are generally used as spreading agents in moisturizers and other liquid and cream skin care and makeup products. Make sure all moisturizers, foundations, and creams that you use have been tested for comedogenicity by an independent laboratory. Look for this information on the product package.

**Q** Which treatment concept is the most important?

**A** *All* of the concepts are important, and failing to use all of them together will not provide the best results. For example, if you use a good oil-control cleanser and daily exfoliant that also kills bacteria, but still wear oily cream-based foundation that clogs the pores, you will "spin wheels" with your treatment progress.

Treating problem skin *must* be thought of as a treatment *program*.

**Q** What is a typical skin care regimen for acne-prone skin?

**A** The morning routine should consist of the following:

- A foaming wash-off cleanser, normally used in the shower with room temperature (not hot) water. The choice of

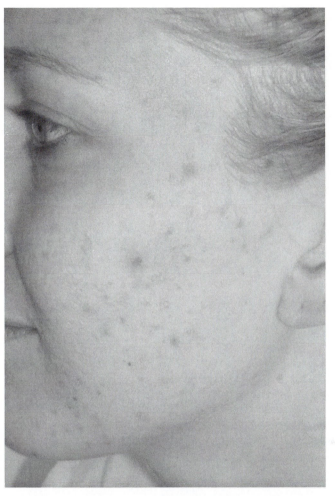

This client had grade-2 acne with many closed comedones, papules, and pustules *(courtesy Mark Lees Skin Care, Inc.)*.

which strength of cleanser should be determined by the severity of the acne, the oiliness level of the skin, and the sensitivity of the skin. People with skin that has acne with many pustules and papules should choose a medicated (with benzoyl peroxide or salicylic acid) wash.

- A low-pH toner, again chosen by the specific skin needs as mentioned above. This toner may contain an antibacterial such as salicylic acid.
- A non-comedogenic sunscreen-moisturizer.

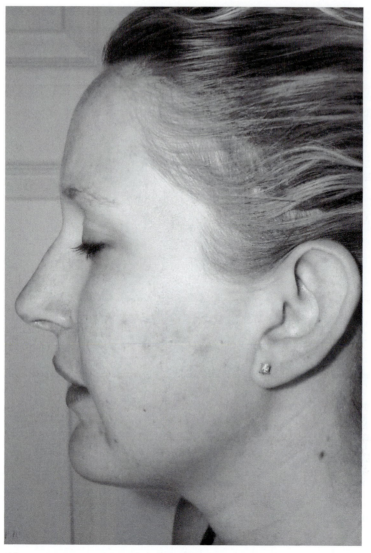

After using a program of alpha hydroxy acid gel, benzoyl peroxide gel, and non-comedogenic products for a 3-month period, this client showed a remarkable improvement *(courtesy Mark Lees Skin Care, Inc.)*.

■ If makeup is worn, it should be completely non-comedogenic.

The evening program should consist of the following:

■ A liquid cleansing milk designed for oily skin to remove makeup. This product should be non-comedogenic and not leave residues. If desired, the foaming cleanser used in the morning can be used a second time.

- Use toner as in the morning.
- Follicle exfoliant treatment—this may be a benzoyl peroxide gel or alpha/beta hydroxy gel or a sulfur-resorcinol lotion. The strength and concentration level of this product should be determined by the severity of the skin problems.
- If a moisturizer is used, it should be a lightweight, non-comedogenic hydrator.
- A non-comedogenic eye crème can be used if needed.

**Q** **What is the best makeup for acne?**

**A** Look for lightweight liquids that have been tested for acnegenicity and comedogenicity. Silicone-based makeup using ingredients such as cyclomethicone are unlikely to cause comedones.

Quick-drying foundations are helpful for oily and acne-prone skin. These makeup products are usually suspensions, which means they separate in the bottle. They must be shaken to be blended before application. They often contain a mild alcohol or witch hazel distillate that causes the spreading agent to evaporate quickly. This eliminates exposure to spreading agents that can cause clogged pores. The evaporation also helps to minimize pore appearance.

Mineral makeup, a powder foundation, is usually acceptable for acne-prone skin as long as it does not contain comedogenic fatty materials to press the product into a compact or to help it adhere to the skin. Check the label carefully to see if any fatty materials are in the powder product. The same would be true for pressed powder and loose powder that is not a mineral foundation.

Blushes should always be checked for D & C red dyes known to clog follicles, as well as pressing agents that can be comedogenic. It is always better to use powder blush instead of crème blush on acne-prone skin. Concealers, highlighters, and other products used on acne-prone facial areas should always be checked for comedogenic testing or ingredients.

**Q** **How long will it take my acne to clear?**

**A** This varies greatly, but, in general, some improvement should be seen in the first 4–6 weeks of treatment, and if the program is followed closely, it should continue to improve over time.

Following the skin care regimen is imperative for improvement. Many programs fail because part or all of the program is dropped or not followed properly. If the skin does not improve, or seems to worsen, a dermatologist should be consulted.

**Q** **Why does acne start at puberty?**

**A** At puberty, young adults begin to produce sex hormones. These sex hormones are responsible for girls developing breasts, developing a figure, beginning menses, and developing the ability to conceive. In boys, hormonal change at puberty is responsible for the voice becoming deeper, growth of body hair, developing a more masculine physique, and the ability to produce sperm.

Male hormones, known as **androgens,** are produced by the testes in males and by the adrenal gland in females. Androgen is an endocrine hormone, meaning it flows directly into the bloodstream. Among other functions, androgen is a stimulant for the sebaceous gland.

When puberty begins and androgens first begin affecting the skin, you may notice pores beginning to appear on the face. This sudden appearance of pore openings is due to the follicles being dilated from the sebum flowing through the follicle canal. The pores begin appearing on the nose, then slowly spreading across the T-zone, including the forehead and chin. Scalp hair may suddenly become oilier, as there are many sebaceous glands in the follicles on the scalp as well.

Androgens work by "switching on" sebaceous glands. Androgens in the bloodstream flow throughout the body, eventually coming in contact with the sebaceous glands. The androgen hormone attaches to a sebaceous cell similarly to the way a spaceship docks at a space station. The hormone then biochemically causes the gland's cells to start producing sebum. The sebum coats over the cell buildup and causes the development of clogged pores and impaction as previously discussed. The sebum may also cause follicle inflammation that may subsequently cause the follicle walls to swell, making it difficult for oxygen to penetrate the follicle. The lack of oxygen sets up the perfect environment for acne bacteria. The eventual result is a comedo or pimple.

It is not unusual to see a young person with comedones and pimples just on the nose or just in the T-zone. The sebaceous glands most often affect the face in the following order: the nose, the chin, the bridge of the nose, forehead, and eventually the cheeks. Pimples and acne lesions are best treated when the symptoms begin. It is important to teach young teenagers how to use the right products, including follicle exfoliants such as alpha hydroxy acids and benzoyl peroxide and other techniques to treat and prevent acne lesions.

**Q** **Why do some people never have acne problems until they are in their 20s?**

**A** Acne is not just a teenage problem. People can have acne problems at any age. Some people continue to have oily skin and acne tendencies into their 40s, 50s, and 60s. In general, however, males are more likely to have problems in their teens and then clear up in their 20s. Females are much more likely to have acne problems well into their 20s and beyond.

Some of this pattern has to do with hereditary blueprints, but most has to do with hormones. Because women have more intricate hormonal processes, the body's glands secrete different amounts of different hormones at different times during the cycle. Such things as birth control pills, illnesses, and events such as pregnancy may also affect some of these fluctuations.

It can also be argued that, in their 20s, women are more likely to wear makeup, which may contribute to the problem if the makeup is comedogenic or acnegenic. Stress also may play a stronger factor for people in their 20s than in their teen years.

**Q**  **What causes pre-period breakouts?**

**A**  About 7–10 days before a woman's period, the body realizes that this cycle's egg will not be used and begins a hormonal process to start the menstruation period. There are a series of hormonal biochemical reactions that take place within the body to accomplish this, and during the process, hormonal fluctuations occur that can stimulate the sebaceous glands. This stimulation can cause inflammation and surges of sebum in the follicle that can result in a pimple or breakout.

**Q**  **Is there anything that can be done to alleviate or prevent premenstrual breakouts?**

**A**  Make sure that you are using a daily follicle exfoliant like an alpha hydroxy/beta hydroxy gel or low-strength (2½%) benzoyl peroxide gel. These chemical exfoliants help to break up existing cellular impactions in the follicle as well as keep cell buildup from reoccurring. This will help keep follicles clear, so if inflammation or sebum surges occur in the premenstrual period, the follicle will be less likely to become occluded, blocking oxygen and creating an anaerobic environment, perfect for the *P. acnes* bacteria to thrive.

Benzoyl peroxide and beta hydroxy salicylic acid are also helpful because they are antibacterials that kill acne bacteria in the follicle.

Use of an overnight spot treatment containing sulfur or sulfur-resorcinol will help to quickly dry up individual pimples.

Having a deep-cleansing facial treatment using galvanic desincrustation with extractions and/or salon alpha hydroxy exfoliation about mid-cycle (15 days before the menstrual period) seems to help some women avoid breakouts.

Women who experience severe premenstrual breakouts every month, even with good skin care, should consult a dermatologist or an endocrinologist. Tests can determine hormonal disorders and treatment may alleviate or lessen the problem.

**Q** **How does stress affect acne?**

**A** It is now well accepted that stress can cause almost any illness or disorder to be worse or more pronounced, and in some cases, stress may totally trigger a biological issue. In acne, though, stress affects hormonal levels, especially in females. In women, much of the androgen or male hormone in the body is produced in the adrenal gland. When stress occurs, the adrenal gland works to produce **adrenaline,** a hormone to cope with stress. It is adrenaline that causes the heart to "rush" when a sudden event happens, such as a near-accident.

When the adrenal gland is in "overdrive" producing adrenaline to cope with a stressful situation, androgens are also being produced in larger quantities, making it more likely for sebaceous glands to be stimulated, more sebum to flow, and more follicles to become impacted and result in a breakout.

If you notice that you tend to break out during stressful times, try to use stress-coping techniques such as exercise, a routine massage appointment, yoga, or meditation to learn to relax. Using your skin care program ritualistically is also a good idea!

**Q** **Can facials help acne?**

**A** Facial treatments can be helpful for people with acne and clogged pores, as long as they are properly performed and accompanied by a good home-care program. If improperly performed, facials can be irritating for acne.

Extraction is beneficial especially in prevention of new pimples if properly performed. This technique helps rid the follicles of impactions that could eventually develop into an inflammatory acne lesion, such as a papule or pustule.

**Q** **What type of facial might be irritating for acne?**

**A** Facials that involve a lot of massage can be irritating for acne. Massage can actually stimulate sebaceous glands, which is not helpful for acne and oily skin types. Facial massage also often involves oily products that can clog the follicles or cause flares of acne. Light–touch pressure point massage performed without massage oils can be relaxing without aggravating acne. Facials that involve a lot of heavily scented products can be inflammatory, as fragrances are well documented to cause irritation, especially in skin that is already inflamed.

**Q** **What should a good acne or oily-skin facial include?**

**A** A good facial for acne-prone skin should include the following:

- Start with a thorough cleansing of the face with a cleansing milk designed for oilier skin.
- A second cleansing using a foaming cleanser may be appropriate for extra oily skin.

- The skin should be thoroughly examined by the esthetician to determine the specific problems with the skin and any treatment that should be avoided.

- A **desincrustation** product will be applied to all areas with clogged pores and impactions. Desincrustation products are alkaline products that help to loosen and break down fatty impactions in follicles to make extraction easier. They may be in fluid or gel forms.

- The esthetician may apply **galvanic current** over the desincrustation product. This current helps to force the desincrustant deeper into the follicles. Galvanic current should not be used on persons with heart issues, epilepsy, metal bone pins or plates, pregnant women, or anyone with questionable health.

- **Extraction** is the removal of debris and impactions from the follicles. It is probably the most beneficial part of a facial treatment for acne and clogged pores, and also the most difficult for the esthetician. Pressure techniques use cotton-covered fingertips, cotton swabs, or instruments called **comedone extractors.** Pressure is applied to the sides of the follicle and, since the impacted sebum has been softened by the use of the desincrustation product, the content of the follicle is expelled. Sometimes, the esthetician may dilate the follicle opening of closed comedones with a lancet prior to extraction to make the extraction easier and safer. (Please note that some state boards that regulate estheticians still do not permit lancet dilation, although more are accepting this as a normal and routine skin care procedure.)

- An antiseptic should be applied after extraction. For acne, this is sometimes an application of a benzoyl peroxide gel. Soothing serum is also often applied. Use of a soothing product after extraction reduces the chances of post-facial breakouts.

- **High frequency current** may also be applied after extraction. This helps to reduce surface bacteria and reduce swelling. Sometimes a serum may be applied prior to application of high frequency, which also helps with penetration of such a product.

- Massage is usually not performed in a facial treatment for acne.

- A clay-based facial mask is often applied after extraction and treatment. This mask will contain an antibacterial such as sulfur. The mask will dry and harden but should not be left on so long that it cracks. Masks that overdry the skin can irritate. Sometimes in more sensitive or irritated skin, a soothing gel-type mask is applied instead of a clay mask. These masks contain soothing agents such as matricaria extract (a type of chamomile), aloe, green tea, or licorice extract. They help reduce redness and hydrate without oils.

- Masks are usually removed with cool cotton compresses or warm (not hot) towels. The compresses are applied to the face and gently pressed to help loosen and wet the mask treatment for removal. This is especially helpful and necessary in removing clay-based masks.

- A toner is often sprayed onto the skin after mask removal. The toner should have a lower pH to help balance the skin's pH at the end of the treatment.

- To finish the treatment, a non-comedogenic, non-greasy hydrating sunscreen is applied.

- It is best not to wear makeup for 2 hours after an extraction treatment. Immediate application of makeup may cause further inflammation. Allowing the skin to have an adjustment period reduces the chances of irritation.

**Q** **How often are extraction treatments recommended?**

**A** Depending on the severity of the problem, it is often recommended that acne facials be performed every 1–2 weeks until the skin is substantially clearer, and then maintain the results with treatments every 4 weeks.

Extraction treatments can be helpful for acne and oily, clogged skin, but they do *not* replace good home care. Twice-daily care at home as previously discussed is extremely important to exfoliate the inside of the follicle to reduce reoccurrence of impactions and prevent flares of acne.

**Q** What about professional exfoliation treatments for acne?

**A** Depending on the type of acne and inflammation, superficial peeling may help or may irritate the skin. Very inflamed acne should not be exfoliated.

It is helpful to use superficial peeling such as 30% alpha hydroxy or glycolic acid exfoliating to help reduce cell buildup and ease in extraction of noninflamed but clogged skin.

The skin should be prepared for 30% alpha hydroxy intensive treatment by using a 10% gel at home on a daily basis. In many cases, a 10% alpha hydroxy gel is a standard part of a home care regimen for this skin type, so most people are already prepared. Microdermabrasion may also be helpful in noninflamed, clogged, nonsensitive skin, but it is not appropriate for inflamed acne.

Alpha hydroxy treatments, performed in series, are often used and helpful to improve the texture and color tone of acne-prone skin that has been successfully cleared prior to the exfoliation treatments.

A good esthetician will be able to determine if and when chemical exfoliation is appropriate in each individual case.

**Q** Does what I eat really affect acne or cause flares?

**A** This is a hard question to answer because there is so much to be learned about nutrition and specifically how it affects the skin.

For many years, the myth that chocolate and greasy foods cause acne has been passed from generation to generation. It has long been believed by the scientific community that what a person ate did not affect acne, with one or two exceptions.

Recent research, however, indicates that there may be correlations in the following circumstances:

- **Dairy products**—In some cases, consuming dairy products may worsen acne. This does *not* affect everyone, so rather than give up all dairy products, try to determine if dairy affects your skin. If you have acne flares and suspect a connection with consuming dairy products, give up dairy products for 3–4 weeks and see if the skin condition improves. If it does, dairy products may have an influence. If you do not see any difference in your skin condition, dairy probably has no effect. The same experiment can work for any suspected food group.

- **High-glycemic foods**—Highly processed, sugar-rich foods have also been rumored over the years to be a possible cause of acne. In a recent study, it was shown that there may be a correlation between a high-glycemic diet and acne. However, questions have been raised because when a diet is changed to low-glycemic, there is often also a drop in dietary fat and an increase in fiber, which might be a factor.

- **High iodide diets**—This has long been thought to worsen acne, but this does not mean that if you eat sushi one night, you will have acne the next day. The level of iodide has to be fairly high for a longer period of time to affect acne conditions. Most cases observed have been in persons taking supplements that were very high in iodide, such as ingested seaweed or algae extract supplements that may be high in iodide content.

The bottom line seems to be that a sensible, balanced diet is probably the best bet, and it is still not established that any particular food rules apply to everyone. There may also be genetic factors that influence how individuals deal biochemically with different foods.

**Q** **Why are dairy foods a problem for some people with acne?**

**A** Most milk comes from pregnant cows, and pregnant cows have many types of hormones and growth factors in their milk to support calf growth. (This is *not* from hormones fed to cows. The presence of hormones in cow's milk is normal.) It is theorized that these hormones and other substances may influence stimulation of the sebaceous glands. The reaction is similar to that of premenstrual breakouts.

**Q** **Does picking make acne worse?**

**A** **Acne excoriée** is the medical term for acne that has been excoriated, which means scratched or scraped. Chronic picking at acne lesions can injure the skin, spread bacteria, and even possibly cause scars.

Acne excoriée is obvious when the skin appears to have acne but, on closer examination, all of the lesions are flat, scraped-looking marks, and sometimes there are scabs on the skin. Another sign of acne excoriée is that the skin rarely has clogged pores or comedones because the patient has also picked them.

Excoriated lesions often are pigmented from inflammation or from exposing the broken skin to sun. This appears as multiple dark round patches on the skin. People with acne excoriée sometimes visit an esthetician or dermatologist complaining about the dark splotches. However, the splotches would not be there if the blemishes had not been scraped. To rid the skin of the pigmented blotches, the patient must stop excoriating the skin.

There can be any number of types of bacteria or other pathogens under the fingernails. Scraping the skin with the nails provides an easy way for these germs to get into the skin and cause an infection, or even to get into the bloodstream.

**Q.** How is acne excoriée treated?

**A** The treatment is to try to stop the patient from picking at the lesions. Some people pick at their skin subconsciously—they are not mindful that they are picking and scratching at the skin. Wearing cotton mitts or lightweight gloves may make them aware of their habit as well as prevent scratching. Wearing sculptured nails also makes them aware, as well as making it difficult to pick.

Estheticians can help the excoriée patient by offering to move up the facial appointment when the patient feels the need to pick. Advising the use of a mask instead of picking may help the problem as well.

Some acne excoriée patients also suffer from mental illness such as obsessive-compulsive disorder and may need the help of a mental health professional.

**Q.** Why do I have red marks for weeks and weeks after a pimple has cleared?

**A** The immune system is responsible for defending the body, including the follicles, from pathogens and foreign invaders. The immune system cells that defend the body reside in the bloodstream and are transported to various sites via the blood. This explains why redness usually accompanies inflammation—the redness is from the blood present in the area. The blood has brought the immune system cells to the area to investigate and defend! When you have a pimple (papule or pustule), the immune cells have fought off the acne bacteria in the ruptured follicle. Blood has engulfed the follicle in the process and blood vessels in the area may have dilated.

Even though the lesion has healed, the blood vessels may still be enlarged in the area. This explains the lingering redness. Normally, the blood vessels will return to normal and the redness will fade in a few weeks. People with light-colored skin, particularly those of Irish or Celtic descent, are more likely to have problems with redness.

**Q** Is there any treatment to speed up the fading of the redness?

**A** Gentle, light-touch massage of the area may help to speed the fading. Treatment with high frequency current or LED light therapy may also be beneficial.

**Q** I have acne-prone skin, but my skin is sensitive and reddens and dries out easily. Are there any special techniques I should use to treat my skin?

**A** Yes. For sensitive acne-prone skin, choose a foaming cleanser that is designed for combination skin. These cleansers contain less detergent than stronger cleansers designed for very oily and acne-prone skin. They are less likely to strip or dry out sensitive skin. Also, make sure all your products are fragrance-free because fragrance can irritate sensitive skin.

Choose lower strength acne products. Benzoyl peroxide gel is usually available in 2.5%, 5%, and 10% strengths. Choose the 2.5%—it is much gentler and is often just as effective for treating acne as the higher percentages. You can also apply it for shorter periods of time. Instead of wearing it all night, leave it on for an hour and rinse it off, or alternate application night by night with a non-oily, non-comedogenic hydrating fluid.

Salicylic acid gel is a different acne treatment and is often used instead of benzoyl peroxide for sensitive, acne-prone skin. If you have only a few lesions, you may want to try an alpha hydroxy/beta hydroxy gel. These, in general, are gentler formulations, as long as the pH is not lower than 3.5.

**Q** I have skin that has many clogged pores, but I rarely have pimples. What would be my best course of treatment?

**A** Many people have oily or combination skin and have problems with clogged pores and comedones, but they rarely have inflammatory lesions (papules and pustules). The best treatment regimen for this skin type is similar to the acne regimen, but less aggressive and we have to worry less about bacteria.

### Morning

- Wash the skin with a foaming gel cleanser containing a gentle cleansing agent such as ammonium lauryl sulfate. Rinse thoroughly with room-temperature water.
- Spray the face with a nonalcoholic toner that contains a hydrating agent. This helps hydrate and lowers the pH after cleansing.
- Apply a coin-sized amount of 10% alpha hydroxy acid gel with a pH of 3.5. Gently massage into all clogged areas until absorbed. Allow to absorb completely.
- Apply a non-comedogenic sunscreen with built-in hydrator. This should be lightweight and thoroughly tested to be non-comedogenic.
- Apply eye cream if desired. This also should be non-comedogenic, because eye cream tends to drift to clog-prone areas of the face such as the upper cheeks.
- If makeup is worn, it should also be non-comedogenic.

### Evening

- Remove makeup with a cleansing milk designed for oily or combination skin. Massage into the skin and remove thoroughly with a room-temperature wet cloth or sponges. Rinse again after removal. If desired, the skin can then be washed with the foaming cleanser as in the morning.
- Repeat toner as in the morning.
- Repeat alpha hydroxy gel as in the morning.
- Apply a blemish-drying lotion to any inflammatory pimples.
- Apply a non-comedogenic hydrator.
- Apply eye cream as in the morning.

Regular extraction treatments by a qualified esthetician will help to dislodge larger comedones and closed comedones.

**Q** **Is there anything that will really shrink pores?**

**A** There is nothing that will permanently shrink pores. Pore size is determined by the amount of sebum flowing thorough the follicle and genetics. Sebum production and follicle structure is hereditary. Scar tissue may also be present from previous acne lesions in the form of "icepick" scars, also often called "open pores" by consumers.

There are treatments that can temporarily minimize the appearance of large pores. Most of these products contain an astringent or alcohol ingredient.

Regular use of an alpha hydroxy acid gel helps to remove debris from the follicles. Removal of this debris and any comedones will help the pores look smaller. This effect is longer-range and generally takes 6–8 months of regular alpha hydroxy gel use to see the effects.

**Q** **I have acne-prone skin, but I am also worried about aging. Can I help reduce the signs of aging without flaring my acne?**

**A** This is a frequent question. Pimples do not understand age and can occur at any age.

The trick here in treating aging in acne-prone skin is to make sure you watch the vehicles or spreading agents of the products you use. As previously discussed, spreading agents may contain fatty materials that can clog or cause acne flares.

You can use all the wonderful smoothing and firming ingredients, but you must make sure that they are in a product that has been thoroughly tested for comedogenicity, and that the product is not *also* intended for alipidic (oil-dry) skin. Many "antiaging" products have rich emollients in them that may be beneficial for dry, mature skin, but they can cause real problems for oily or acne-prone mature skin.

Alpha hydroxy acids (which are helpful in remedying both clogging and signs of aging) in a gel form, lightweight hydrators, non-comedogenic sunscreens, peptides, or anti-oxidants in water-based serums are all perfect for helping mature, acne-prone skin.

Estheticians who are familiar with comedogenicity can be helpful in making choices for these skin types.

**Q.** **How important is cleansing for acne-prone skin?**

**A** Acne is not caused by dirt or dirtiness. However, it is important to control the excessive sebum that is associated with acne-prone and clogged, oily skin.

Ideally, a foaming, rinseable cleanser should be used once or twice a day. If makeup is worn, it should be removed using a cleansing milk designed for oily skin, so it does not leave clogging residues.

The strength of the cleanser will vary with the severity of the oiliness or acne condition. Gel or foaming cleansers are traditionally made in combination, oily, extra oily, and acne-medicated versions.

**Q.** **When should I go to a dermatologist?**

**A** You may go to a dermatologist at any time. Often estheticians and dermatologists work together or have referral relationships.

All of the treatments we have discussed so far in this chapter are over-the-counter (OTC) treatments or treatment products available through a licensed esthetician. Estheticians should always refer to a dermatologist when they suspect that their client needs medical help.

When you have acne that does not respond to all of the treatments we have discussed, a dermatologist should be consulted. Acne skin that has a lot of pustules, indicating more substantial infection, should also be seen. This condition often needs oral antibiotics as well as topical care.

**Q** How does medical treatment for acne differ from over-the-counter or esthetic treatment?

**A** Medical treatment of acne is, in general, much stronger than over-the-counter treatments. It also has more side effects, which is why it must be administered by a medical doctor.

Dermatologists often prescribe prescription-strength topical retinoid (vitamin A derivatives) topical drugs for acne. These are all strong **keratolytics** (peeling agents) to remove and flush debris from follicles. The mission is the same as we have already discussed, but the product (drug) is much stronger. Retin-A, Tazorac, and Differin are commonly prescribed retinoids. Other non-retinoid topical peeling drugs prescribed are Azelex (azelaic acid) and Sulfacet (sulfacetamide). These should not be used with other nonprescription peeling agents unless approved by the dermatologist.

Topical antibiotics are often prescribed to accompany the keratolytic. They include erythromycin and clindamycin (Cleocin-T).

Oral antibiotics are prescribed in more severe or non-responsive cases. They include drugs such as tetracycline, minocycline, and erythromycin.

**Cystic acne** is a severe form of acne in which the skin forms deep pockets of infection. Cystic acne must be treated by a dermatologist. **Accutane** is an oral prescription retinoid used to treat cystic acne. Accutane can be an effective drug for cystic acne but has many possible severe side effects.

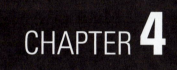

# CHAPTER 4

# Sensitive, Redness-, and Allergy-Prone Skin

**Q** What is sensitive skin?

**A** There is no real medical definition of sensitive skin, but sensitive skin is skin that is more reactive to treatments and is also more likely to experience irritation than normal (nonsensitive) skin. Sensitive skin definitely has barrier function defects, allowing nerve endings to be exposed to nerve irritants. Some persons with sensitive skin may have more reactive immune responses and higher than normal neurological (nerve) reactivity. Some experts believe that sensitive skin is created by over-exfoliation and overexposure to stimulating skin care products.

People with sensitive skin have problems with **subjective symptoms** such as burning, stinging, and itching. Subjective symptoms are symptoms that are felt but not visible. These are symptoms of neurological reactivity. **Objective symptoms** are visible and often measurable. Redness and flaking are two objective symptoms of sensitive skin.

**Q** Is sensitive skin hereditary?

**A** Possibly, but what is definitely hereditary is skin structure associated with genetics. Redheads with light, fair skin and blue or green eyes (Fitzpatrick Type I skin) have thinner skin than someone who is of Mediterranean descent. Mediterranean skin is Fitzpatrick Type IV skin and is thicker skin less likely to have barrier function issues. Persons who are of western European descent such as Irish, Scottish, British, or Celtic are more likely to have thinner sensitive skin.

A thinner epidermis allows closer exposure to nerve endings and blood vessels. These skin types are much more sensitive to sun, heat, and cold. Again, because of the thin skin layers, the barrier lipids are generally not as plentiful, making it easier to have barrier function damage. This damage can allow penetration of irritants that lead to inflammation and redness. A damaged barrier also allows **transepidermal**

**water loss (TEWL),** commonly known as dehydration, which can cause dryness, flaking, itching, and stinging.

**Q** **Why does sensitive skin turn red easily?**

**A** The blood vessels in Fitzpatrick Type I skin are closer to the skin surface hereditarily. Any inflammation or even heat or embarrassment will cause dilation of facial blood vessels. In thinner skin, this blood rush is visible because the skin is both thin and light in color.

   The immune system, which is within the blood system, is easily excited in sensitive skin. Whenever the immune system responds to an invader or an inflammatory substance, the area will flush with blood as an immune function. This turns the skin red immediately, and the skin will stay red as long as inflammation exists.

**Q** **Why does thin skin constantly look pink?**

**A** Even without inflammation, fair-skinned people will appear to have pink tones to their skin due to the blood being close to the surface. The lack of pigment in this skin coloring also makes redness more obvious.

**Q** **Does the condition of the barrier function affect redness?**

**A** Very much so! An impaired barrier function allows penetration of potential irritants through the skin surface, causing inflammatory responses from the immune system through the bloodstream. Whenever an irritant enters the skin, the immune system responds, sending blood to the area as an immune defense strategy. This shows up on the skin as redness.

**Q** **Can improving the barrier function decrease redness?**

**A** Absolutely! Not only will a better barrier function reduce redness, it will help reduce sensitivity, as well as burning, tingling, or itching. Hydration will be visibly improved, making skin look smoother and less flaky.

Here are the rules for better barrier function in sensitive skin:

- Use a low-foaming or nonfoaming cleanser, such as a cleansing milk. Find one designed for sensitive skin that is fragrance-free and has been dermatologist-tested for irritancy. It may also contain soothing ingredients to reduce redness. Foaming cleansers contain detergents designed to remove excess sebum. Because the sensitive skin is thinner, it generally has less sebum. The detergent begins removing lipids in the barrier instead!
- Be careful with ingredients that enhance penetration including acid exfoliants, propylene glycol, or volatile alcohols (which may be acceptable to use on other skin types). Make sure to check that toners are designed and tested for sensitive skin.
- Be careful with mechanical exfoliants, such as scrubs or microdermabrasion, that can also affect the barrier function.
- Use products that contain lipid replacements to help patch and enhance the barrier function. These include sphingolipids, phospholipids, fatty acids, and cholesterol.
- In severely sensitive skin, products that contain petrolatum or silicones may be used to create a false barrier on top of the skin. This can help the barrier to restore itself naturally, assuming all insults to the barrier have been stopped.
- Sun exposure causes barrier lipid reduction, especially in sensitive skin.

**Q** What are the basic concepts for treating sensitive skin?

**A** There are several basic concepts to reduce redness and sensitivity:

- Avoid all well-known irritants and allergens. This would include all fragrances, essential oils, products that contain drying or volatile ingredients such as isopropyl or SD alcohol, menthol, mint extracts, citrus extracts, drying clay masks, and other products that stimulate the blood flow.

- Avoid any product that strips the skin or leaves it feeling tight and dry. This includes many washes and soaps. Scrubs should be used cautiously, if at all.
- Avoid heat and sun. Both of these can dilate blood vessels in thinner skin and inflame the skin.
- Keep the skin as cool as possible.
- Use a sunscreen daily. Although this is advice for any skin type, it is especially important for Fitzpatrick Type I and sensitive skin. Zinc oxide is a good, less-reactive ingredient that is sensitive skin–friendly.
- Use a nonfragranced moisturizer daily. This should be selected for your specific skin type (oily, dry, combination, etc.) and should be designed for sensitive skin.
- Be careful with highly acidic products. Alpha hydroxy acids can be helpful for sensitive skin but should be used carefully. Consulting with a qualified esthetician is a good idea.
- As discussed in the previous question, protect and reinforce the barrier function of the skin. Faulty or damaged barrier function is a hallmark characteristic of all inflamed skin.
- Choose products designed for sensitive skin and tested for irritancy potential in an independent laboratory.
- Talk to your esthetician or dermatologist if you have trouble finding the right product program for your skin.

**Q** Are there specific ingredients helpful for sensitive skin?

**A** The following ingredients may be helpful in calming or preventing redness in sensitive skin:

-  Decyl glucoside is a gentle cleansing agent that cleanses without stripping the skin. Look for it in cleansers for sensitive skin.

- Lipid ingredients help repair or reinforce the barrier function by "patching holes" in the "mortar." When the barrier is fully intact, irritants, including some cosmetic ingredients, are unable to penetrate the skin, resulting in less reactivity, less redness, and less inflammation. In addition, the skin hydration level is increased and protected. This makes the skin look less red and smoother on the surface. Lipid complexes can be mixed into sunscreens, moisturizers, serums, masks, eye creams, and other products. Look specifically for sphingolipids, glycosphingolipids, phospholipids, ceramides, fatty acids, and cholesterol. These ingredients are almost always used in combination to mimic the actual lipid mix in the natural barrier function.
- Antioxidants such as grapeseed, green tea, or matricaria extracts neutralize free radicals and help to squelch inflammation and redness. They are also beneficial to help prevent premature skin aging.
- Soothing ingredients include the above antioxidants, plus antiredness ingredients such as stearyl glycyrrhetinate, bisabolol, azulene, and sea whip (elizabethae) extracts.

**Q** I get really red after I get my lip waxed and sometimes stay red for hours. Is there something I can do to avoid this?

**A** Make sure that a body temperature or cold wax is being used for epilation. This will initially help because of reduced heat, and will also be less irritating when removed from the skin.

The skin should be cleansed prior to waxing, and then a light application of powder before application of the wax will allow the wax to adhere to the hair, but not the skin. A soothing antiseptic lotion should always be applied after the waxing treatment. Avoid makeup application for at least 2 hours.

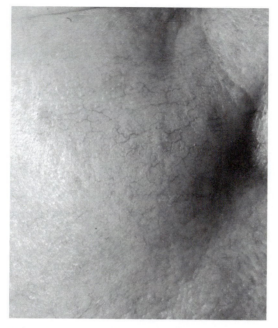

Telangiectasias—distended capillaries.

Use of cool compresses after the waxing may also soothe the irritated wax area.

 **Are "broken" capillaries really broken?**

A These little red blood vessels found in different areas of the face are actually distended or dilated capillaries, known medically as **telangiectasias.** They are often erroneously called "broken" capillaries. The capillaries are not broken or there would be bruising present.

The red color indicates that they are arterial capillaries. This blood is oxygenated and coming from the heart to the skin. Venous capillaries, going back to the heart, are blue in color.

**Q What causes distended capillaries?**

A Distended capillaries, also known by the European term **couperose,** are found primarily in lighter skin colors.

There is definitely a hereditary tendency to capillary distension in lighter skin types of western European descent.

The distended capillaries can be caused by constant friction, such as abrasive action from facial tissue or repeatedly blowing the nose. Distended capillaries are often found on the sides of the nose.

High blood pressure, excessive sun, excessive alcohol consumption, facial injuries, rosacea, and smoking have all been linked and are believed to be causes of distended capillaries.

Many women experience distended facial capillaries during pregnancy, but most of these seem to spontaneously clear after delivery.

People with distended capillaries should avoid any source of heat exposure, sun exposure, and stimulation to the facial skin. Distended capillaries are best treated by a medical professional using laser or intense pulse light (IPL). They also can be treated with an electric needle. The treatments are generally performed in a dermatologist's or plastic surgeon's office.

**Q** **My doctor says I have rosacea. What can you tell me about rosacea?**

**A** **Rosacea** is a **vascular** (involving the blood circulation) disorder that results in diffuse redness, facial swelling, acne-like papules and pustules, distended capillaries, and, in some cases, enlargement of the nose.

Rosacea is hereditary and is especially predominant in persons of light-colored skin and western European descent.

There are four subtypes of rosacea:

Erythematotelangiectatic rosacea presents as diffuse redness in the nose and cheeks and sometimes the forehead. It may have a grainy texture and feel dry. It is sometimes referred to as "dry rosacea" by estheticians.

Papulopustular rosacea has large acne-like papules and pustules with surrounding redness.

Ocular rosacea affects the eyes and eyelids. Styes, thickening and reddening of the eyelid skin, and redness of the eyes are frequent symptoms.

Phymatous rosacea is the subtype of rosacea that causes swelling of the nose and growth of the cartilage in the nose. The famous comedian W. C. Fields had **rhinophyma,** which is the term used to describe the enlarged nose of rosacea. Men are more likely to have phymatous rosacea, but women are more likely to have rosacea in general.

**Q** **What can be done to help rosacea?**

**A** There are many **triggers,** a term used to describe factors that cause **flushing,** or sudden reddening of the facial skin from sudden increased blood flow. Flushing leads to **flares,** when skin with rosacea begins having obvious symptoms and inflammation.

Whenever the skin is flushed with blood, a biochemical within the skin called **vascular growth factor** is

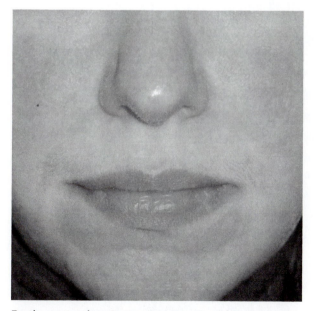

Erythematotelangiectactic rosacea—"dry rosacea"
*(courtesy National Rosacea Society).*

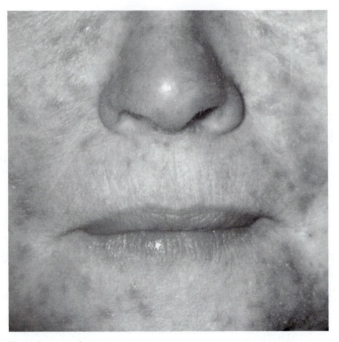

Papulopustular rosacea *(courtesy National Rosacea Society)*.

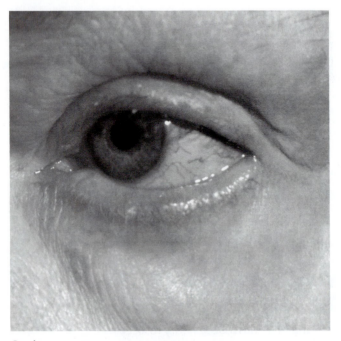

Ocular rosacea *(courtesy National Rosacea Society)*.

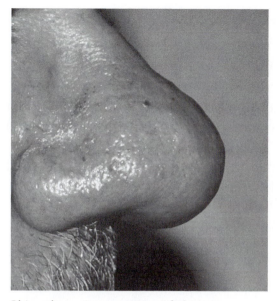

Rhinophyma is a symptom of phymatous rosacea
*(courtesy National Rosacea Society)*.

released. This triggers expansion and growth of new blood vessels, further increasing the chances of flushing and flares. This is how rosacea worsens over time if flushing is not controlled.

Avoidance of the following triggers is important for persons who have rosacea:

- Heat exposure of any type is a major factor in flaring all types of rosacea;
- Sun exposure, especially without sunscreen protection;
- Stimulating skin treatments or products containing ingredients such as peppermint, menthol, and essential oils;
- Aggressive massage or friction of any type;
- Overdrying the skin or overdrying masks;
- Acids and exfoliants, depending on the strength and frequency of use;
- And other factors that promote increased blood flow to the skin.

**Q** My nose gets really red when I drink red wine. Is this rosacea?

**A** It might be, but this can only be confirmed by a physician, preferably a dermatologist. Reddening of the skin when alcohol is consumed is one of the classic signs of rosacea. Wine contains tannins, alcohol, and sulfites. All of these can cause blood vessel dilation.

Other foods that have been implicated in rosacea flares are coffee, other hot beverages, citrus fruits and juices, and spicy food. Not all foods listed affect every rosacea case. If you have been diagnosed with rosacea by a physician, you should watch for foods that may be correlated with flares in your particular case and then avoid those foods.

**Q** My rosacea seems to flare when I exercise. Does this make any sense?

**A** Yes, this is a commonly shared observation of rosacea patients. Exercise raises the heart rate and stimulates circulation of the blood. This can cause flushing of the facial skin, which can lead to a flare. The keys here are heat and increased blood flow.

Try to exercise inside where there is air conditioning or swim at a time of day when the sun is not intense. The keys here are to avoid heat, sunlight, and raising the body temperature—all of which can lead to flushing and subsequent rosacea flares.

**Q** Why does heat have such a strong effect on sensitive skin?

**A** Heat dilates blood vessels, increasing blood flow and redness. In sensitive skin, the blood and nerve endings are both closer to the skin surface, making them more susceptible to stimulation.

Persons with sensitive skin should avoid hot baths, hot facial steam treatments, saunas, sun exposure, and prolonged exposure to hot weather. Exposure to any heat source can aggravate sensitive skin.

Because many people with sensitive skin also have Fitzpatrick Type I coloring, they are more likely to sunburn, get sun damage, and develop skin cancer. They must wear sunscreen at all times when outside and should make sunscreen a part of their daily skin care regimen.

**Q** **What type of skin care program should I use if I have rosacea?**

**A** Skin care for rosacea is more about what not to do than what to do. Avoiding stimulants and abrasives or anything that increases heat is important. Avoid any product that strips or overcleans the skin.

The following steps are generally recommended for rosacea and other sensitive skin:

- Use a gentle, nonstripping, nonfragranced cleanser. For oilier rosacea or oilier sensitive skin, a mild foaming cleanser is good. For dry rosacea or dry sensitive skin, use a nonfoaming cleansing milk. Make sure all products are fragrance-free, because fragrance can aggravate sensitive skin or rosacea.
- Use a nonalcoholic toner. This toner should be free of astringents or stimulants such as alcohol, menthol, or citrus extracts.
- Alpha hydroxy exfoliants should be used carefully on sensitive skin or skin with rosacea. AHAs are believed to help rosacea as long as they are not used when the rosacea is flared. If possible, choose an AHA serum with added soothing agents. Consulting a skin care professional is a good idea when choosing an AHA product for sensitive skin.
- There are antiredness serums that may reduce redness and soothe rosacea flushing. These serums contain soothing ingredients such as elizabethae (sea whip)

extract, matricaria (chamomile) extract, or licorice extracts. They may also contain antioxidants such as green tea or grapeseed extracts.

■ Sunscreens used for rosacea or sensitive skin should contain a physical screen such as zinc oxide or titanium dioxide, which help to bounce sunrays away from the skin, preventing heating of the skin surface. Sunscreens for rosacea should be fragrance-free, lightweight, and non-comedogenic.

**Q** **What are medical treatments for rosacea?**

**A** Metronidazole is a topical antibiotic often prescribed for rosacea. Originally designed to treat yeast infections, metronidazole has an anti-inflammatory effect on rosacea. Metronidazole is marketed under the name Metrogel or Metrocreme and also as Noritate. Another prescription drug used for rosacea is Finacea, containing azelaic acid, and a third drug is Sulfacet, containing a sulfur compound called sulfacetamide. In severe flares of rosacea, secondary bacterial infections can occur, and oral antibiotics such as tetracycline may be prescribed.

Laser treatments or intense pulsed light (IPL) treatments are sometimes used to treat telangiectasias (dilated capillaries), and sometimes **ablative** (tissue-removing) lasers are used to actually remove surface skin tissue in severe rosacea cases. This removal of tissue also removes blood vessels, slowing the progression of the disease.

At this time, there is no cure for rosacea. The key is to keep rosacea from progressing by keeping the skin from flaring.

**Q** **What causes skin allergies?**

**A** Skin allergies are largely hereditary; however, they can occur at any time in life. Allergies are individualized and do not affect everyone.

An **allergy** is the body's immune system rejecting a particular substance. The substance could be a food, airborne substance, or a topical or cosmetic ingredient. The skin is triggered to respond to skin **allergens** by reddening, swelling, developing **urticaria** (hives), and other biochemically induced responses to the offending substance.

**Q** **Are there skin care ingredients that frequently cause allergies?**

**A** The most frequent allergen in the cosmetic and skin care world is fragrance! Fragrance is added to many products to make them more appealing to the senses.

It does not matter if the fragrance is natural or synthetic. Essential oils are a frequent cause of skin care allergy.

In general, the following people should avoid fragranced products:

- People who have a lot of skin allergies have redness-prone skin;
- People who tend to have skin reactions;
- And people who have been diagnosed with rosacea or other inflammatory skin conditions.

Other common skin allergens are the following:

- Color agents
- Lanolin
- Nail products
- Sunscreens
- Hydroquinone (skin lightening ingredient)
- Preservatives, especially those that release formaldehyde

**Q** **Are natural products less likely to cause allergies?**

**A** No! This is a common mistaken belief.

Most allergens contain some sort of protein. Natural extracts, because they come from living plants, often contain proteins. Peanut, milk, and egg allergies are examples of frequent protein-based allergies.

**Q** **What is the difference between an allergic and an irritant reaction?**

**A** Allergic reactions are rejections of a substance by the body's immune system. Irritant reactions are skin reactions usually caused by exposure to an irritating chemical that causes a caustic or peeling effect on the skin.

Allergic reactions only affect certain people, while irritant reactions can affect anyone. For example, only certain people may be allergic to peanut oil, but everyone will be irritated by a strong acid or overuse of a peeling acne product. Irritant reactions are usually only isolated to the area of application, while allergic reactions can affect larger areas or the whole body.

Substances that cause irritant reaction may not cause a reaction if the dosage or frequency of application is reduced. Substances that cause allergic reaction will react regardless of dosage or frequency of application.

**Q** **Can you exfoliate sensitive skin?**

**A** Sensitive skin is often sensitive because it has been over-exfoliated. Red, inflamed skin should never have mechanical or chemical exfoliation performed, nor should an exfoliation product be used at home while the skin is irritated or inflamed.

Skin that tends to be sensitive can be carefully exfoliated using a mild granular product that is buffered with moisturizing or emollient ingredients. The product should feel slightly grainy but not sharp or rough to the touch. Exfoliants for more sensitive skin are often thicker emulsions to avoid over-contact with the exfoliating granules.

Chemical exfoliants such as alpha hydroxy acid serums or creams can be used if the skin is not red and inflamed. These products should be no more than 10% alpha hydroxy acid with a pH no lower than 3.5. Using a product designed and tested to be used on sensitive skin is the best choice.

Sensitive skin may not tolerate exfoliation as often as normal skin even if using a weaker exfoliant. Discontinue use immediately if redness or inflammation occurs and persists. For example, some people with sensitive skin can use an AHA product every other night, or once a day instead of twice a day. A good rule of thumb with sensitive skin is, "when in doubt, don't!"

**Q** **Does what I eat help or hurt my sensitive skin?**

**A** Some people who have skin allergies may have respiratory or food allergies. There is no particular food to avoid for everyone. Allergies vary greatly from person to person.

People who have rosacea may have to avoid red wine, alcohol, spicy foods, caffeine, hot beverages, or citrus fruit. These foods are known to cause flushing and rosacea flares in more than a few rosacea patients. Not everyone has reactions from all these foods.

Besides eating a well-balanced diet that has plenty of antioxidants and omega-3 fatty acids, there is no known special nutritional trick for helping sensitive skin.

**Q** **Are there facial treatments that should be avoided for sensitive skin or clients with rosacea?**

**A** The following treatments should be avoided on sensitive or rosacea skin:

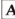 Heat treatments of any kind, including hot steam. If steam is used it should be focused far enough away

from the face so that the skin does not feel heat. Cool steam from an ultrasonic steamer or a Lucas spray device is a better choice.

- Exfoliating treatments including scrubs, microdermabrasion, or chemical exfoliation should only be used if the skin is not inflamed and the esthetician is familiar with the sensitivity level of the particular person's skin.
- Hot masks such as paraffin
- Hard-setting clay-type masks that dry the skin
- Essential oils or fragranced treatment
- Any treatment that stimulates blood flow
- Strong or excessive massage. Light, slow massage or light fingertip tapping is usually fine.

The following is a suggested facial treatment for sensitive skin:

- Lightly wet the skin. Gently apply a nonfoaming cleansing milk designed and tested for sensitive skin to the face with gentle circular movements. Gently massage in all facial areas.
- Using a soft damp cloth or dampened cotton pad, remove the cleansing milk thoroughly.
- Apply a nonfragranced hydrator or serum designed for sensitive skin to the face.
- Apply cool steam from an ultrasonic steamer for 5–6 minutes. If an ultrasonic steamer is not available, apply cool, wet compresses across the face for 5–6 minutes.
- If an esthetician is performing the treatment, light and gentle extractions of comedones can be done at this point.
- Apply a mild, nonalcoholic, nonfragranced toner on a cotton pad, or gently spray onto the face with an atomizer.
- Apply a nonfragranced soothing moisturizing fluid and gently massage the face.

- Apply a gel-based mask with soothing ingredients such as matricaria extract, green tea, or licorice extract. This gel mask will hydrate the skin well, without causing drying or inflammation.
- Thoroughly remove the mask with cool, wet, soft cloths or cotton pads. Do not cause excessive friction on the face while removing the mask. Applying a wet compress before removal helps to loosen and soften the mask for easier removal.
- Apply a moisturizing sunscreen for sensitive skin.
- Makeup should be avoided for at least 2 hours after treatment.

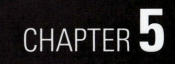

CHAPTER **5**

# Dry Skin

**Q** **What causes dry skin?**

**A** Dry skin is caused by water or moisture escaping from the surface layers of the skin. This is commonly known as **dehydrated** skin, or medically as **xerosis.** Water escapes from the skin into the dry air.

The dehydrated skin suffers from dryness, flaking, tightness, itching, and sometimes stinging and burning. Lines and aging symptoms look worse when the skin is dehydrated.

Much like the dryness of the surface of a desert, the skin can develop cracks and fissures in the surface. It can also become inflamed and red.

Esthetically, dehydrated skin forms fine lines easily due to surface cells being "deflated," lacking water that normally makes the surface smoother and more supple. The skin may even appear to have the look of being covered with plastic wrap. The slightest touch or gentle pinch causes multiple fine lines and wrinkles. Well-hydrated skin does not respond this way.

Aging symptoms look worse when the skin is dehydrated. The lack of moisture in the skin surface makes the skin appear rough, or even flaky, and can be rough to the touch. Wrinkles look deeper and more numerous, and elastosis is more obvious. Because of the pileup of dead dry cells on the surface, the skin can have a dull, even gray-looking, appearance.

There are many factors associated with dry skin:

- **Lack of natural sebum protection** allows easy escape of water because there is no protective layer of sebum on the surface of the skin to shield against water evaporation.
- **Skin with impaired or poor barrier function** results from insufficient lipids between the epidermal cells. These gaps in the barrier function allow deeper moisture to escape from the skin.

- **Poorly protected or poorly moisturized skin** can easily become dehydrated, especially when other factors also play a part. Sometimes people do not use any moisturizer or protectant, and some make the wrong choice of moisturizer for their skin type.
- **Washing the skin too frequently** can deplete the skin of its protective sebum or, if the skin is already dry, begin stripping lipids between the cells that comprise the barrier function.
- **Low humidity** creates a demand for more moisture in the air. Unprotected skin easily loses water by osmosis to the air.
- **Poor health and medication side effects** can also contribute to skin dryness.

**Q** Is there more than one type of dry skin?

**A** Estheticians refer to skin as being either dehydrated or **oil-dry.** Any skin can become dehydrated if exposed to enough stripping of the outside protective levels. First the protective sebum layer is stripped, and then the barrier function lipids are affected.

A windburn or mild winter frostbite on the cheeks is dehydration. The flaking caused from sunburn is also severely dehydrated skin. Also referred to as **water-dry** skin, dehydration can also occur from overusing peeling agents or overcleansing.

Oil-dry or **alipidic** skin is skin that is not producing enough protective sebum to prevent surface dehydration. Alipidic skin is characterized by a lack of visible pores. This indicates that there is little sebum being produced by the sebaceous glands in this skin since the follicles are not dilated.

Sebum normally provides a fatty layer on the surface of the skin to help protect against dehydration. If a skin is alipidic, this layer of sebum is not sufficient to protect the skin surface from water evaporation and eventual additional damage to the barrier function.

**Q** **Is barrier function important in dry skin treatment?**

**A** Yes! Lack of barrier function can cause or worsen dry skin. It is the barrier function—the complex of fatty material *between* the epidermal cells—that keeps moisture from escaping the epidermal cell layers. If the barrier function is impaired, it cannot provide this protection.

The best ways to protect the barrier function include the following:

- Use a good protective moisturizer daily. Choose one that is right and comfortable for your skin type. This will help shield the skin against water evaporation and add a layer to protect the barrier.
- If you have a tendency to become dehydrated easily, look for moisturizers that contain lipids to supplement the barrier function. These include glycosphingolipids, phospholipids, ceramides, fatty acids such as linoleic acid, and cholesterol.
- Do not over-wash the skin or use cleansers than are stronger than what your individual skin needs. This removes too much protective sebum and possibly lipids that form the barrier function.
- Do not over-exfoliate the skin. Over-exfoliation can strip barrier function causing dehydration as well as inflammation.

**Q** **Does skin get drier with age?**

**A** In general, yes. As we age, our cell renewal cycle in the epidermis slows. It is the cell renewal cycle that creates the intercellular lipids that comprise the barrier function. As the renewal cycle slows, so does the production of these important protective lipids. The cycle is also affected by cumulative sun damage over the years.

The skin also produces less sebum as we age. Less sebum on the skin surface means less protection. The skin can become dehydrated easier, especially when exposed to stronger soaps or detergents.

Diseases such as thyroid disease and diabetes can also cause or worsen dry skin. Many diseases can cause dry skin, or the medications used to treat certain diseases cause dry skin as a side effect.

The hormone estrogen also influences dry skin. After menopause, this hormone decreases substantially in the bloodstream. This can affect skin dryness and decrease the production of collagen in the dermis.

**Q** **Does dry skin cause wrinkles?**

**A** Dry skin can certainly make wrinkles look worse. Dryness can cause fine lines and wrinkles, but deeper wrinkles, as well as elastosis, are mainly caused by facial expression and cumulative sun exposure. However, the lack of moisture in the surface can accentuate both wrinkles and elastosis, as well as make the surface of the skin look rough and dull.

Dehydration can make aging skin look older, and the appearance can be improved by the consistent use of good moisturizers; it must be accepted that these effects are temporary and that the wrinkles and elastosis are really caused by years of unprotected sun exposure. This damage still exists under a well-moisturized, sun-damaged skin and will reveal itself quickly if moisturization stops.

Good moisturization can make any wrinkle look better, but moisturizer must be used consistently to constantly plump the surface skin to smooth the appearance. Moisturizer alone does not have long-term affects on existing wrinkles but possibly can help prevent new wrinkles.

When the skin is dry, and the barrier function is impaired, the skin is easily inflamed. Inflammation causes a chain of biochemical reactions that lead to collagen and elastin breakdown. If the skin is protected and the barrier function is intact, inflammation is much less likely to occur. So, in this way, moisturization and skin protection can help prevent wrinkles!

Estheticians use enzymes and mild AHAs to remove dead, dry surface cells, making the skin look smoother and feel softer. They also use intensive moisture treatments to plump the surface cells and restore barrier function. All of these can make a wrinkled or sagging skin look better, at least temporarily. Home care must be performed routinely to maintain the results.

**Q** What are basic concepts in correctly treating dry skin?

**A** Dry skin can be easily treated, but frequency and consistency of treatment is extremely important:

- Dry skin needs surface protection in the form of a moisturizer containing protectants or emollients. This is especially important for skin that is alipidic and not providing adequate protection naturally. These ingredients form a shield or protective layer on top of the skin, preventing dehydration and allowing the barrier function to eventually repair itself. They are also often the spreading agent in the moisturizer. The concentration of emollient in the moisturizer will vary with the dryness level of the skin. Skin that produces little sebum will require a richer moisturizer. The richness of a moisturizer is determined by the amount of emollient ingredients in the formulation.
- Moisturizers must contain water-loving **humectants,** also known as **hydrophilic agents** or **hydrators,** that help to attract water and bind the moisture to the cells and between the epidermal cells.
- Humectants and emollients work together in a moisturizer. Humectants attract the water and emollients guard against its evaporation from the skin. Different

combinations of concentrations of humectants and emollients create different formulations with different thicknesses, spreadability, and heaviness. A product with little emollient, designed for dehydrated skin that is also somewhat oily or combination skin, will be a lightweight and thinner lotion or fluid. The more alipidic the skin, the more it is necessary to have more emollient concentration in a moisturizer. A product designed for alipidic skin will be much heavier due to the higher emollient content and will most often take the form of a cream.

- Lipid ingredients in products help to "patch" and supplement barrier function. These are not the same as emollient ingredients that lie on top of the skin. The lipid ingredients in a formulation go between the cells to supplement and fill the gaps between epidermal cells.

- Promote gentle stimulation of the cell renewal cycle. Gentle exfoliation using mild alpha hydroxy acids helps promote cell renewal, improve hydration, and improve natural production of intercellular lipids for the barrier function. Exfoliation also rids the skin of dried surface cells, improving moisturization penetration and effectiveness, making the skin look smoother and less wrinkled.

- Moisturizer must be used routinely to treat and prevent dry skin. Generally it should be used at least twice a day. Hand moisturizer may be used multiple times a day, depending on how often the hands are washed.

- Skin should not be stripped by using soaps, cleansers, or peeling agents that are too strong for the specific skin type.

- As with most skin problems, prevention is the best treatment. Using a good moisturizer right for your skin every day and taking care to avoid exposures that create dry skin are two ways to prevent skin from becoming dry.

**Q** What is the specific role of emollient ingredients in the treatment of dry skin?

**A** Emollients lie on top of the skin in a protective layer, shielding the skin from moisture loss. They act as substitutes for a protective sebum layer for skin that is alipidic.

Emollients such as petrolatum or mineral oil are good guarding agents for severely dehydrated skin, allowing the skin to rebuild its natural barrier function over time. These agents are excellent for dry skin "in crisis" because they completely block moisture loss and do not cause allergy or irritant issues. They can be used alone for more severe cases or in moisturizing products for less dry skin or moisture maintenance.

Natural oils such as jojoba, sunflower seed oil, safflower oil, or borage oils contain natural fatty materials helpful in protecting the skin and also supplementing the barrier function. These oils are much more comfortable to use than petrolatum, but they do not provide the same occlusion. They are more appropriate for skin that *tends* to be dry, instead of severely dry skin.

The fatty materials in the barrier function are often used in formulations for dry skin; however, they are included to help patch the actual barrier, not to lie on top of skin to protect it from further dehydration.

Silicone-based ingredients such as cyclomethicone, dimethicone, and cyclopentasiloxane provide good daily but lightweight and non-pore-clogging protection. They are all also non-comedogenic, so they do not clog pores if they are used on combination or acne-prone skin.

**Q** What are commonly used humectants for treating dry or dehydrated skin?

**A** Humectants are used for treating dehydrated skin, whether or not it is also alipidic. Humectants attract water and bind it to the skin. Emollients keep it from escaping. Commonly used humectants include sodium PCA, glycerin, sodium hyaluronate, hyaluronic acid, sorbitol, and propylene or butylene glycol.

Products designed for oilier or combination skin will have a good amount of humectant, but less emollient.

**Q** **Why does dry skin get worse in the winter months?**

**A** Dry air and exposure to cold and wind can make dry skin much worse in the winter. The low humidity in the air creates an osmotic condition in which the water levels in the surface of the skin easily evaporate into the air.

Walking outside and exposure to cold, dry outside air can create not only dry but also chapped and irritated skin, mainly on the face and hands.

Indoor heat in the winter further dries the air, again creating a condition that robs the skin of moisture. The skin is exposed to dry air 24 hours a day in the winter, inside and outside.

**Q** **Is there anything I can do to avoid winter dryness?**

**A** Dry skin can be flaky and itchy, and in the winter months, this is commonly known as winter itch.

The best treatments are the following:

- Make sure you apply a good moisturizer every day. The best time to apply a moisturizing product is immediately after a bath or shower, before the skin is completely dry.
- Do not bathe more than once a day.
- Take shorter showers or baths. Lingering in the bath can deplete surface oils.
- Take cooler or room-temperature showers. Hot showers and baths strip more natural protective sebum from the skin and can inflame skin that is already dry.
- Avoid traditional soaps and highly foaming cleansers that tend to strip protective lipids and can strip lipids in the barrier function if the skin is already dry.

- Moisturizers that contain alpha hydroxy acids help to build more natural lipids in the epidermal barrier function.
- Consistency is important in both treatment and prevention of dry skin. The skin must be cared for every day!
- If you visit a skin therapist, there are a number of dry skin treatments for body skin available, including paraffin and seaweed treatments. These can give the dry skin a moisture "boost," but daily home care is still imperative.

**Q** **Do room humidifiers help dry skin?**

**A** Yes. Room humidifiers create moisture-laden air that does not dry the skin. Skin still should be treated with a moisturizer, as it will be exposed to dry, cold air outside.

It even helps to expose water to the air without a humidifier. Leave open bowls of water in your home, especially in the bedroom. They will evaporate into the air, raising the humidity level. You must remember to refill the bowls routinely—you will be surprised how fast the water evaporates!

**Q** **Does flying in a plane make skin drier?**

**A** Many people, including flight attendants, complain of dryness after flying. The recycled air is like being in a dry heated house, and the pressurized cabin may contribute as well.

Use a good moisturizing protectant before you fly. If you are on a long flight, reapplication may be needed.

**Q** **Why does my skin seem so dry and tight when I get out of the shower?**

**A** Wet skin dries out quickly as moisture on the outside of the skin quickly evaporates into dry air. As previously mentioned, apply a moisturizer immediately after taking a bath or shower to seal this moisture in, rather than allowing it to evaporate. Also, avoid using stripping soap or heavy foaming cleansers when showering or bathing. Switch to a less-aggressive cleanser for the winter months.

**Q** **Why do soaps seem to make my dry skin worse?**

**A** Many soaps have high pHs that strip the skin of its protective surface barrier. Continued use of high pH soaps can further irritate and strip barrier lipids.

**Q** **Are there special cleansers for dry skin? What makes them special?**

**A** Cleansers for dry skin contain less detergent or surfactant ingredients than those for normal skin. They foam less, indicative of the lower concentration of these cleansing agents. Because of the lesser concentration, they remove less protective sebum.

Secondly, cleansers for dry skin often contain emollient or fatty ingredients that help to buffer the contact of the cleansing agents with the skin. Some even leave a residue of emollient on the skin after use.

Facial cleansers for dry skin are either low-foam or no-foam. Emollient-type cleansers can remove makeup and surface dirt without stripping the skin of its natural protection. Some cleansers for dry skin are produced with special methods that use a smaller amount of emulsifier or no emulsifier. Emulsifiers are surfactant-like ingredients that keep emulsions properly mixed. Large amounts of emulsifiers in products can also further dry skin that is already dry.

Because dry skin can also be sensitive, it is best to avoid fragranced products for this skin.

**Q** **Do bath oils help dry skin?**

**A** If you are using bath oils to relax, they are better than using bubble bath, which can dry the skin further. Bath oils coat the skin, which helps to seal in moisture, but may also coat the skin and prevent water penetration during the bath. It is probably more beneficial to apply a good moisturizer at the end of your bath.

**Q** **What kind of moisturizer should I choose for dry skin?**

**A** For body skin, it is generally a good idea to choose a lotion that contains a good combination of humectant and emollient. Avoiding fragrance is a good idea, especially if the skin is already dry and irritated. Body moisturizers that contain an alpha hydroxy acid, usually glycolic or lactic acid, may be helpful in not only moisturizing but also ridding the skin of surface dried dead cells, flakiness, or ashiness.

Body creams are heavier than lotions but are also more difficult to use, and they may feel heavy or oily for some time after application. Body oils are good lubricants, but they do not contain humectants.

For facial skin, the choice should be based on the oiliness level of the skin. There are moisturizers formulated for dry, combination, and oily skin. They will vary in heaviness and emollient content. Choose one that feels right for your skin and provides enough moisture so that you do not need to reapply the product. Also make sure you choose one that does not make you feel oily.

If you have breakout-prone skin, choose a hydrating fluid that has been tested to make sure it does not clog pores.

**Q** **Are there ingredients or products that I should avoid for dry skin?**

**A** If you have dry skin, you should avoid the following:

- Products containing drying or volatile alcohols such as isopropyl or SD alcohols. Do not get these mixed up with fatty alcohols such as cetyl alcohol or stearyl alcohol, which are actually emollients.

- Products that have extremely high or low pHs. This would include strong low pH (lower than 3.5) exfoliants or astringents and some cleansers or desincrustant products that have pHs higher than 6.0. These products may be fine for normal to oily skin, but not for dry skin.
- Fragranced products, and especially heavily fragranced products, may be irritating to dry skin whose barrier function is already impaired, making this skin more vulnerable to irritation and inflammation.
- Highly foaming, stripping washes have already been discussed. These products strip the dry skin of its natural protection.
- Rough scrubs or exfoliating products.

**Q** What is a good step-by-step home care program for dry skin?

**A** The following is a typical daily program for dry skin. For specific products for an individual skin, an esthetician should be consulted.

**Morning care:**
- Wet the skin with tepid water. Apply a gentle nonfoaming or low-foaming cleanser and gently massage across the face. Remove with tepid wet soft cloths or wet cotton pads.
- Spray the skin with a nonalcoholic toner specially designed for dry skin. This should contain a hydrating agent such as butylene glycol. Gently pat the skin dry. Do not overdry.
- Apply a moisturizer designed for your degree of dryness. For oily or combination dehydrated skin this may be a fluid or lotion. For drier skin it will be a creamier product. For most skin types, a built-in sunscreen in the moisturizer will help skip an additional step. For severely dry skin, a separate moisturizer may need to be applied prior to sunscreen.

- Apply an eye cream to eye areas.
- Apply makeup as desired.

**Night care:**
- Apply a makeup-removing nonfoaming cleanser designed for dry skin directly to the face. Massage gently in circular movements. Using a wet soft cloth or cotton pad, gently remove the makeup thoroughly. If the skin is not completely clean, repeat the procedure.
- Apply toner as in the morning.
- Apply any serums, which might include peptides, antioxidants, AHAs, or other conditioning agents.
- Apply a hydrating product appropriate for your skin type. This, again, may be a fluid or a cream. Massage this thoroughly into the skin surface. Make sure you use enough of this product to thoroughly cover the face.
- Apply eye cream as needed.

**Q** Why does dry skin itch?

**A** Dry skin has exposed gaps in the barrier function, making nerve endings more exposed. When surface cells dry, they become brittle and itchy. When the skin is scratched, these cells are removed and the skin becomes inflamed—and can even become red and itchier!

Most skin itching can be controlled by the routine use of a good moisturizer. Some moisturizers contain anti-itch ingredients. For severely itchy skin, a product containing cortisone may need to be used. These should only be used for brief periods of time, and if the skin continues to itch severely, a dermatologist should be consulted.

**Q** Does it help to exfoliate dry skin?

**A** As long as it is done gently, mild exfoliation gets rid of dead dry surface cells and promotes cell turnover, which helps produce lipids for the barrier function. Exfoliating scrubs containing beads made of smooth polyethylene or hydro-genated jojoba oil are good choices.

Some of the most effective moisturizers contain alpha hydroxy acids, which serve as humectants and as exfoliating agents. AHAs help to rid the skin of dead, dried-up cells and smooth the skin surface, improving the esthetic appearance as well.

**Q** What type of facial treatments can help dry skin?

**A** Professional facial treatments can be helpful for dry skin, but they must be performed routinely, such as every week or two, to have any lasting effect. They certainly do not replace a good home care program. Dry skin must be cared for 24 hours a day to treat or prevent dryness.

Occlusive treatments are helpful for dry and dehydrated skin. This would include alginate (seaweed) mask treatments, paraffin masks, collagen "blankets," and other masks that form a solid sheet that can be removed in one piece.

Before application of the occlusive mask, a hydrating fluid or cream is applied and massaged into the skin. The mask treatments create an occlusion that forces the hydrating agents into the surface of the skin.

**Q** Do steam treatments help dry skin?

**A** Steam treatments can be helpful and soothing for dehydrated skin, but steam treatment must be followed by application of moisturizers or masks to be effective. In addition, after the facial treatment, proper moisturization and good skin care habits must be followed to have lasting results.

**Q** Are peels helpful for dry skin?

**A** As long as the skin is not cracked or inflamed, light exfoliating peels such as enzymes or mild alpha hydroxy acid peels can help accelerate cell turnover and remove dry, dead cells from the surface. This will give the skin a boost, and moisturizing treatments will be more effective.

Dry skin can easily be over-exfoliated, and emphasis should be placed on using mild exfoliating products and being careful not to use them too often.

Again, peels do not replace good daily care of the dry skin.

**Q** **Is massage helpful for dry skin?**

**A** Massage can be very helpful for dry skin. Massage increases blood flow to the skin and can help stimulate sebaceous glands to produce more sebum. Massage can also help hydrating products absorb into the skin surface more efficiently.

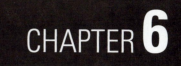

# CHAPTER 6

# Sun Care

**Why is it important to wear sunscreen every day?**

A  Sun is the number-one enemy of the skin.

- Sun exposure is the number-one cause of premature aging of the skin.
- Sun exposure is the number-one cause of skin cancer.
- Sun exposure is the number-one cause of cancer because there are more cases of skin cancer than any other form of cancer.

Besides avoiding sun exposure, using sunscreen on a daily basis is the number-one skin cancer prevention technique, and the number-one premature skin aging prevention technique.

Many people only use sunscreen when they go the beach. They erroneously think that when the skin has direct intense sun exposure is the only time sunscreen needs to be used. Sun damage is cumulative, and while it is important to use sunscreen when in direct sunlight, such as a trip to the beach, the real damage comes from *cumulative* sun damage over a lifetime.

Sun exposure causes the formation of free radicals in the skin. Free radicals are wild oxygen-based atoms or molecules that are unstable and desperately need to be stabilized. What will stabilize these wild radicals are electrons, which the radical atom steals from important structures in the skin such as cell membranes and cellular DNA. When the DNA is altered, it changes the "blueprint" for cell replication. When this happens, there is a biochemical potential for the beginning of cancer.

Further, these radicals cause a domino effect of biochemical inflammatory reactions that lead to the production of self-destruct enzymes that destroy collagen, elastin, and hyaluronic acid in the skin. Cumulative destruction of these vital skin components leads to symptoms of what we think of as aging: wrinkles, loss of elasticity (sagging skin), and rough-textured skin. This damage may not show up for years, but eventually the cumulative effects of sun exposure will result in wrinkles, bad skin texture, sagging skin, and likely skin cancer and abnormal growths.

**Q** Why do I need a sunscreen if I am not outside?

**A** Think about a basic workday. You get in your car to go to the office. You park your car and walk across the parking lot. You go into your office and sit by a window while you work.

When you get off work, you walk through the parking lot, drive home, walk to get your mail by the street, walk your dog, play with your kids in the yard, and sit on your back patio and have a glass of wine.

You are outside quite a bit. Multiply that exposure time by 7 days a week, 52 weeks a year, times 20 years! How much sun exposure is that?

Additionally, UVA rays from the sun go through glass. So, you are getting UVA exposure while in your car and while sitting by your office window.

This is called **ambient sun exposure.** It is not deliberate, but these short exposure times over the years can add up to a lot of free radical activity, and a lot of sun damage. The easiest way to prevent this is to get in the habit of applying sunscreen to all exposed areas of your body (don't forget your neck, including the back of your neck, arms, and hands!) every morning.

**Q** I have naturally dark-pigmented skin. Do I need to wear a sunscreen every day?

**A** If you have dark skin, your skin has a higher Fitzpatrick scale rating, which means your skin is naturally more resistant to sun exposure and sunburn. However, you should still use a daily sunscreen to prevent eventual inflammatory damage, premature aging, and damage that could still eventually lead to skin cancer. Secondly, people who have darker skin types are generally more susceptible to hyperpigmentation and dark skin splotching. Wearing an SPF-15 daily sunscreen will help prevent this type of hyperpigmentation.

**Q.** **When should children begin using sunscreen?**

**A** Children should be carefully shielded from the sun beginning at birth. Infants should have sunscreen applied when outside as prescribed by their pediatrician. Young children may have allergy problems with sunscreen ingredients, and parents should get advice from their doctor.

Children should be taught to apply sunscreen daily as a basic health habit, just like brushing their teeth or bathing. They should be taught how to effectively apply sunscreen and that application of sunscreen is a part of swimming or going outside. Habits established for children at a young age make a huge difference when they are adults.

**Q.** **What is the difference between UVA and UVB sunrays?**

**A** The sun projects light in a spectrum. A certain area of that spectrum reaches the earth and can affect skin. The two types that affect the skin in a negative way are the ultraviolet A and B rays.

Ultraviolet B (UVB) rays are short rays that penetrate the epidermis to the basal layer. UVB rays cause sunburn and are believed to cause the majority of skin cancers. Ultraviolet A (UVA) rays are longer, more deeply penetrating rays that affect the dermis, and they are believed to cause the most damage to the dermal structure of the skin and may be most responsible for DNA damage and melanoma, the most deadly form of skin cancer. UVA rays, as previously mentioned, can penetrate glass windows.

One easy trick to remember: UV<u>B</u> for burning, UV<u>A</u> for aging!

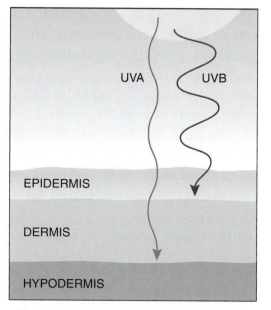

Ultraviolet A and B rays affect different levels of the skin.

**Q** How do sunscreens work?

**A** Active ingredients in sunscreen work by absorbing UV rays and neutralizing them, or by physically reflecting the rays away from the skin.

**Absorbing sunscreen ingredients,** also sometimes wrongly referred to as chemical screens (which is incorrect; all sunscreens are chemicals), absorb and neutralize UV rays. In doing so, they release the energy as heat. While this does not bother most people, the heat may cause problems for people with rosacea or sensitive skin.

The following ingredients are absorbing sunscreen active ingredients: avobenzone (Parsol 1789), octinoxate, octisalate, octocrylene, oxybenzone, ecamsule (Mexoryl), homosalate, padimate A, and padimate O.

**Physical sunscreen ingredients** work by reflecting or scattering rays from the skin. There are only two FDA-approved physical sunscreen ingredients: titanium dioxide and zinc oxide.

Zinc oxide and titanium dioxide are sometimes referred to as "chemical-free" sunscreens, another erroneous term because they *are* chemicals. It would be more correct to call them "heat-reflecting."

The physical sunscreens are considered to be less irritating than the absorbing screens because they disperse heat rather than absorbing the light and heat energy. They are also less likely to cause allergic reactions or inflammation than their absorbing counterparts. These physical agents are considered to be some of the most effective sunscreen agents, physical or absorbing.

The problem with physical sunscreen ingredients is that they often have to be suspended in thicker spreading agents to be applied evenly on the skin. This creates usage issues and sometimes a thicker, stickier product, which many consumers do not like. They also have a tendency to have a white, powdery appearance when used alone.

Many companies have remedied this problem by mixing some of the absorbing ingredients with some of the physical sunscreen ingredients. This creates a more cosmetically acceptable product that is much lighter and user-friendly and still allows an effective and less-irritating product.

**Q** **What does *broad-spectrum* mean?**

**A** A sunscreen that is broad-spectrum filters both UVA and UVB rays. As discussed earlier, different sunscreen ingredients filter or reflect different parts of the UV spectrum. The goal is to screen as much of the spectrum as possible.

To screen a larger portion of the spectrum, chemists often mix ingredients that filter different parts of the light spectrum.

- UVB filters include octinoxate, octisalate, homosalate, octocrylene, padimate A, and padimate O.
- UVA absorbers include avobenzone and ecamsule.

- Oxybenzone absorbs a combination of UVB and some UVA.
- Zinc oxide and titanium dioxide reflect most of both sections of spectrum.

**Q** **What does *SPF* mean?**

**A** **SPF** stands for *sun protection factor.* Represented by a number, SPF measures how long you can stay out in the skin without getting a sunburn. If you go out in the sun without sunscreen and normally would burn in 30 minutes, an SPF of 4 would theoretically allow you to stay out four times as long, or 2 hours, without getting a sunburn.

Many scientists believe that the concept of SPF is scientifically outdated because it measures how long it takes for clinical inflammation to appear. We now know that the skin becomes inflamed and cellular damage can appear long before the skin turns red. It is now believed that the width of the spectrum filtered by a sunscreen is a better measure of how good a sunscreen is.

At the time of this writing the FDA has proposed a new labeling system to rate the amount of UV filtered, and for the first time will test UVA exposure as well. It may take time for this labeling to appear on sunscreen products.

**Q** **Which is the best SPF to prevent damage?**

**A** Most dermatologists and skin scientists believe that a sunscreen with an SPF of 15 or above is adequate for most people. Higher SPFs may be more appropriate for people who expect to be in direct sunlight for long periods of time.

**Q** **Do higher SPFs filter more of the spectrum of UV light?**

**A** Only slightly. The difference between an SPF-15 and an SPF-30 sunscreen is about 4% more light filtered. The higher the SPF, the less the spectrum filtered increases.

**Q** What is the difference between a sunscreen and a sunblock?

**A** The FDA used to allow companies to call products containing physical sunscreen ingredients sunblocks. The term *sunblock* is not permitted in the current law. All sunscreen products must now be referred to as sunscreens.

**Q** Has global warming and the thinning of the ozone layer made UV exposure worse?

**A** Yes. The ozone layer has traditionally filtered out much of the spectrum of rays from the sun. Since the ozone layer has thinned, more UV rays reach the earth, making it more important than ever to wear sunscreen every day.

**Q** What type of ray is used in tanning beds and booths?

**A** UVA rays are used in tanning equipment because UVA rays only cause burns in large doses but still cause an immune response resulting in a tan. Remember that a tan is caused by the skin trying to shield itself from harm!

**Q** Is it okay to use a daily sunscreen that is also my moisturizer?

**A** This is one of the best ways to practice effective sun protection. Find a moisturizer that meets your moisturizing needs (a good weight for your skin type, the right thickness, and a comfortable product that meets your beauty needs as well) that is also an SPF 15 or higher broad-spectrum sunscreen.

It is certainly scientifically possible for a moisturizing product to double as a sunscreen. Most people do not need to use a separate moisturizer during the day.

**Q** What should I look for in a good sunscreen?

**A** To review some points we have already discussed, a good sunscreen should do the following:

- Be easy to use on a daily basis. Ideally, it should also serve as a moisturizer. This product should be individualized to suit your skin type, age, moisture level, and individual conditions and sensitivities.
- Be at least an SPF 15.
- Be broad-spectrum, shielding against both UVA and UVB rays.

**Q** Are antioxidants effective sunscreens?

**A** Antioxidants may be helpful in inhibiting free radicals and inflammation due to sun exposure, but they are *not* sunscreens.

Often, antioxidants, including vitamins and botanical extracts, are mixed into sunscreen formulas, after-sun preparations, and serums and other products intended for sun-damaged skin. Although they may help with appearance-related problems from short-term and long-term sun exposure, they provide no protection against sun exposure.

**Q** Some makeup foundations have sunscreen in them. Is this enough protection?

**A** The problem with makeup that contains sunscreen is that the amount of makeup applied may vary greatly from person to person. Heavy application of a makeup product may provide enough product to protect the skin, but light or partial applications may not provide enough to give the protection desired.

If a combination sunscreen/moisturizer is used prior to applying makeup that also contains sunscreen, this does not add to the SPF of the sunscreen. If a sunscreen/moisturizer has an SPF of 30, applying a makeup product with an SPF of 8 does not combine to give an SPF of 38. The SPF would be the highest of the products applied—in this case, an SPF of 30.

**Q** **Should I choose a water-resistant sunscreen?**

**A** Water-resistant sunscreens are good choices if you anticipate a day of swimming or excessive sweating. They are good choices for children over six years of age who are enjoying a day at the beach or pool. Children under six should seek advice from their pediatrician regarding sunscreen choices due to allergy tendencies in young children.

Water-resistant sunscreens tend to be much heavier in texture and oil or emollient content to repel water from the skin. They are often not a good choice for acne-prone skin, as the heavy emollients used in these products may worsen acne or clogged pores.

There is no such thing as a completely waterproof sunscreen. Eventually they will wash off the body. By law, sunscreens making a water-resistant claim must be tested to document that the sunscreen product is still effective after 40 minutes of exposure to water. If the sunscreen makes a "very water resistant" claim, the product must be effective after 80 minutes of water exposure.

**Q** **Is there a difference between sunscreens intended for the face versus the body?**

**A** Sunscreen intended for the face is generally lighter weight in emollient and texture than that intended for the body. Facial sunscreens are often intended to be used with makeup over them. Body sunscreens may be water resistant, while facial sunscreens are not usually water resistant.

Sunscreens designed for the face may also be more likely to contain antioxidants, soothing agents, and other conditioners.

**Q** How much sunscreen should I use?

**A** An average-size person should use one ounce of sunscreen to cover the body with one application. This is the amount that would fit in a typical shot glass, or about ¼ of a standard 4 oz sunscreen bottle.

Sunscreen should be applied at least 30 minutes prior to sun exposure to allow the sunscreen time to absorb into the skin surface. Applying sunscreen once the skin is overexposed and inflamed can actually add to the skin inflammation.

**Q** How often should I reapply sunscreen?

**A** If you are in direct sunlight, the sunscreen should be reapplied every 2 hours, and it should be applied more often if it is not waterproof or you have extremely sun-sensitive skin. Sunscreen should be applied after any time you have been swimming or excessively perspiring.

Sunscreen worn to the office on a typical day without excessive direct sun exposure does not need to be reapplied.

**Q** Do sunscreens expire?

**A** Yes. Sunscreens are regulated as over-the-counter (OTC) drugs in the United States. They are required to be stamped or marked with an expiration date, and they should not be used after the expiration date. Sunscreens should be stored in a cool, dry place, not in the hot trunk of a car! When on the beach, sunscreen should be kept in a cooler if you have one. Otherwise, cover the package with a towel when in the sun.

**Q** Are some people allergic to sunscreens?

**A** Occasionally, someone is allergic to a specific sunscreen ingredient. Because the same sunscreen ingredients are used in so many different formulas on the market, it may seem that the person is allergic to many sunscreens, but it is because they keep trying different ones with the same active ingredient to which they are allergic.

PABA, a good UVB sunscreen used for years, caused enough allergic reactions to gain it a bad reputation, and it has been omitted from most current formulas. Products containing zinc oxide or titanium dioxide definitely cause less irritation, but often these ingredients are mixed with absorbing screen ingredients that are more likely to cause allergies.

Try to determine which ingredient causes allergies for you by checking labels and isolating which ingredient is consistently present in the products that cause reactions for you. Most people can find a group of sunscreen ingredients that they can use without allergy problems.

**Q** **Does cloudy weather make sun less intense?**

**A** Only slightly. This is why meteorologists issue a **UV index** every day in the morning weather report. This index factors in the time of year, proximity to the sun, and atmospheric conditions of a local area in order to determine how much sun is reaching the earth. Pay attention to this index, especially when planning outdoor activities.

Many people will still get sunburns and sun damage on overcast days, erroneously thinking that the sun is not as intense due to cloudiness. Clouds can cut about 20% of sunlight reaching the earth, but rays can still be damaging—there are just not as many. Even in a rainstorm during daylight hours, UV is hitting the earth.

Wearing a broad-spectrum sunscreen every day helps keep you prepared for weather variations that may affect UV intensity.

**Q** **Are you less likely to get sunburn in the winter?**

**A** Only because you are less likely to spend time outdoors! The sun can be just as intense in the winter. Many people are surprised to get a sunburn during their first skiing trip. Not only are they in direct sun on a mountain, but light is bouncing off the white snow and hitting them from a second angle! Dry, cold air and wind can further dry the skin, making the sunburn even more uncomfortable.

*Anytime* you are outside, regardless of time of year, you should wear a good broad-spectrum sunscreen.

**Q** **Are there "safer" times of the day for outdoor activities?**

**A** Yes. The sun is at its peak at noon. It is best to avoid outside sun exposure between 10 a.m. and 3 p.m. Pay attention to the UV index for the day as predicted by meteorologists. Again, proper sun protection and using sunscreen properly can minimize damage and chances of sunburn.

Heat during summer months also can cause excessive sweating and is more likely to effect sunscreen efficacy in the middle of the day. If you are anticipating sweating while participating in outdoors activity, make sure you are using water-resistant sunscreen and reapplying as necessary.

**Q** **Does clothing provide any protection?**

**A** Lightweight cotton clothing usually worn during hot weather provides little protection. It is possible to get sunburned through a T-shirt.

There is specially made clothing now available that has measured SPFs. These clothes are specially designed to reflect light and are still lightweight enough for hot weather. You can find these sun-protective clothing at many sporting stores.

In general, wearing white or lighter colors when in direct sun reflects light and produces less heat. A hat and good sunglasses are also important and helpful to protect eyes from sun damage and prevent squinting that can cause or accentuate wrinkling. Hats and caps prevent damage as well, especially in people with thin hair. Scalps can get sunburned, too, and skin cancers are often found in the scalp.

**Q** Is there any way to get a "safe" tan?

**A** There is no such thing as safe tanning. All unprotected cumulative sun exposure causes damage to the skin that can lead to skin cancer and premature skin aging.

**Q** What about "sunless" and spray tans? Are they safe? How do they work?

**A** Sunless tanning and spray tans both contain an ingredient called **dihydroxyacetone,** which causes keratin proteins in epidermal cells to darken. It is not a real tan involving biological melanin production.

Many improvements have been made in these products in the last few years, and there are specialty items for just the face. Many salons now offer spray tanning or sunless tanning applications as a service.

Sunless tanning is safe, and it is certainly safer than exposing skin to the sun to achieve a tan.

The one caveat is that some people erroneously believe that the dark color is actually a tan, and make the mistake of believing that they now have natural protection against sunburn. Although the darkening does make the skin look tanned, it does not eliminate the need for daily sunscreen use and proper sun protection when outdoors.

**Q** How should the skin be treated if it is sunburned?

**A** Minor sunburn should be treated with cool baths and avoidance of any treatment or product that exfoliates, stimulates, or strips the skin of moisture. Stay inside in a cool environment. Topical soothing agents include cooled aloe vera gel, cool plain (not fruit or frozen) yogurt, or even an over-the-counter (OTC) hydrocortisone lotion. Do not reexpose the skin to more sun!

After the skin has cooled down, a lightweight moisturizer can be applied to make the skin more comfortable.

Topical anesthetics may cause allergic reactions and generally should be avoided. If the skin is "bubbling" or if the sunburned person is feeling faint, dizzy, nauseous, or has other illness symptoms, he or she should be seen immediately by a physician.

**Q** **Are there products you can apply after sunning to minimize damage?**

**A** The best treatment is to avoid sun exposure in the first place! Topical moisturizer can minimize the appearance of peeling and dryness, but it will *not* prevent peeling. Application of antioxidant serum after sunning may help prevent damage but is better applied *before* sun exposure (along with a sunscreen).

There is, unfortunately, no after-sun product or treatment scientifically documented to undo the real and long-term damage done from sun exposure.

# CHAPTER 7

# Dark Spots/ Pigment Problems

**Q** What causes dark splotches on the skin?

**A** There are various reasons why the skin might have dark splotches, but most are caused by **hyperpigmentation**—the melanocytes in the skin have overproduced melanin in the areas of the splotches.

Remember from the earlier chapter on skin function (Chapter 1) that melanocytes are pigment-producing cells present in both the lower epidermis and the upper dermis. The melanocytes are stimulated by sun exposure to produce melanin by "injecting" developing epidermal cells with particles containing melanin called melanosomes. When the pigment is produced in an even fashion, a tan is produced.

When the melanin is produced in an uneven way, or certain areas overproduce melanin, dark splotches or uneven pigment appears. Sometimes this hyperpigmentation will fade naturally as the skin cells shed through the cell renewal process. If the skin is damaged from sun, this hyperpigmentation can be chronic.

**Q** What makes the skin produce more melanin?

**A** There are several causes for hyperpigmentation:

- Sun damage from excessive and cumulative sun exposure
- Hormonal imbalances and pregnancy
- Genetic skin coloring and race
- Injuries and inflammation
- Certain types of disease
- Side effects of some medications

Probably the biggest factor in hyperpigmentation is chronic and cumulative sun exposure. Hyperpigmentation is a definite symptom of sun damage or dermatoheliosis, the dermatological term for skin that has suffered damage from cumulative and excessive sun exposure.

**Q** How is splotching a part of aging skin?

**A** Beautiful, evenly colored skin is one of the characteristics of young and healthy skin. One of the most frequent signs of sun damage to appear is uneven skin coloring, primarily seen on the face, neck, and chest. Sun-related, dark, splotchy hyperpigmentation can affect not only the face but also the body. It can be present in any areas of the skin that have been repeatedly exposed to the sun. On the body, it usually shows up first on the hands and arms.

Uneven pigment or **solar mottling** is often the first symptom of cumulative sun damage to appear. This can occur as early as the late teens or early 20s, but it usually appears in the late 20s or early 30s. In older skin, the skin can become mottled and almost leather-colored. This looks even worse when it is accompanied by sun-induced wrinkles and rough skin texture.

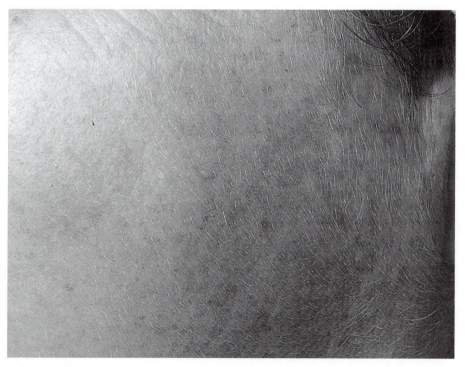

Solar mottling.

The overproduction of melanin in sun-damaged skin is likely to be related to the melanocytes being "stuck in overdrive," trying desperately to protect the skin from the sun exposure.

**Q** **Is hyperpigmentation more of a problem for males or females?**

**A** Because so many pigmentation problems are related to hormone fluctuations and disorders, females are much more likely to have problems with hyperpigmentation. Males can certainly also have problems with hyperpigmentation, but these are primarily related to sun exposure and sun damage.

**Q** **What is a pregnancy mask? Do you have to be pregnant to have one?**

**A** The second most frequent reason for hyperpigmentation is an imbalance of hormones that signal the melanocytes to produce more pigment. This is a common problem for women using birth control pills or other forms of hormonal therapies, and some pregnant women. Hyperpigmentation associated with hormonal influence is known as **melasma.**

Sun exposure may make the symptoms of melasma worse, and it may be worse in women who already have significant sun damage before having hormonal imbalances. *Pregnancy mask* is another term for melasma, but specifically melasma that occurs in the pattern of a mask affecting the forehead, cheeks, chin, and upper lip. This pattern can be strong and distinctive or occur in only certain of these facial areas.

It has been estimated that about 70% of all pregnant women have some form of melasma during pregnancy, but hormonal imbalances can cause pregnancy mask or melasma in women who are not pregnant. Rarely, it also occurs in men.

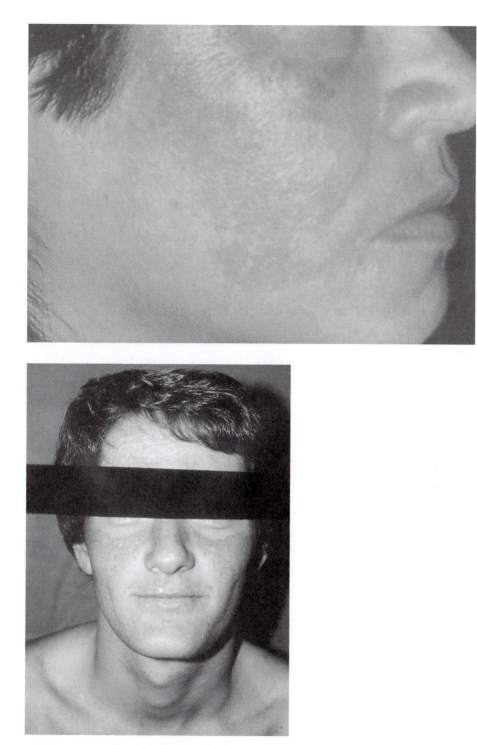

Melasma caused by hormonal imbalances *(courtesy Timothy G. Berger, M.D.)*.

In many women, the melasma spontaneously resolves after the birth of the baby. Some women have lingering melasma problems, though, and these may require treatment.

**Q** **Is heat a factor in dark spots?**

**A** It is believed that heat can stimulate melanocytes, especially in skin with strong tendencies to hyperpigmentation. This has been observed often in cases of melasma, where the skin was protected by high SPF broad-spectrum sunscreen yet still experienced darkening from exposure to heat in the hot weather.

Heat may also be a factor in post-inflammatory hyperpigmentation, especially in Fitzpatrick skin types IV to VI.

**Q** **Is there a hereditary factor in hyperpigmentation?**

**A** Yes. Just as skin color is genetic, tendencies for hyperpigmentation can also have a genetic connection.

**Q** **Is dark skin more likely to have a problem with hyperpigmentation?**

**A** Yes. Dark skin types (Fitzpatrick types IV–VI) are much more likely to have problems with hyperpigmentation. This includes black skin, Asian skin, dark Hispanic skin, and Middle Eastern skin tones.

**Q** **Why do I get dark spots where I have had pimples?**

**A** Many skin types tend to have hyperpigmentation after a pimple, a scrape, or minor injury. This is known as **post-inflammatory hyperpigmentation,** also known as **PIH.** The inflammation that has occurred in the area of the pimple or injury has triggered melanin production as an immune response. In many cases, PIH fades over time

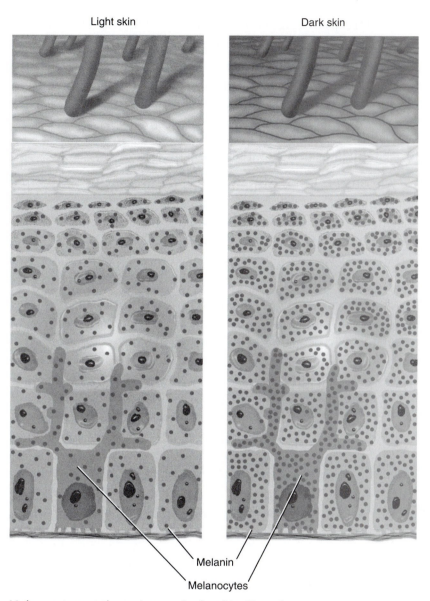

Light skin

Dark skin

Melanin

Melanocytes

Melanocytes produce pigment in the skin. Note the more numerous melanosomes in darker skin.

as the epidermal cells are replaced. Unfortunately, acne often tends to be chronic and may produce chronic PIH in the area of breakouts. PIH in acne-prone skin occurs frequently in skin of color.

The problem that causes the response is the acne. When the acne is treated and brought under control, the PIH will resolve. However, people who get PIH tend to get it easily and from any kind of inflammation to the skin.

**Q** **Can picking at my skin cause dark spots?**

**A** Absolutely! Scraping and scratching at pimples cause inflammation, which in turn causes PIH. This picking is known dermatologically as acne excoriée. Secondly, picking at the skin may cause scratches and injuries that may pigment more easily if the scratched skin is exposed to sun after the injury.

Professional extraction of comedones and impactions is the best way to avoid chances of PIH from acne lesions, although in some skin types this may occur even with proper professional extraction.

Chronically scratching at eczema and other itchy skin conditions can also cause PIH, darkening the skin in the area of the condition.

Darker skin, as mentioned previously, is more likely to have problems with PIH than lighter skin types.

**Q** **What can I do to avoid getting spots where I have had pimples?**

**A** As previously mentioned, avoidance of picking or scraping at pimples will help prevent inflammation and therefore PIH. The best way to prevent these splotches is to treat the acne so that pimples are prevented. Regular (daily) use of a benzoyl peroxide wash, 2.5% benzoyl peroxide gel, or alpha/beta hydroxy acid gel will help to flush follicles of debris that causes the impaction that eventually becomes a pimple. This should be used even in areas of the face where there are no pimples currently present, as the follicles must be flushed in all areas of the face to prevent new pimples. Even when the skin is clear in acne-prone skin, microcomedones—the beginning of clogged follicles—are constantly forming under the skin due to hereditary factors. Daily use of an alpha/beta hydroxy gel or mild benzoyl peroxide gel will keep this follicular debris from accumulating.

Alpha hydroxy acids and benzoyl peroxide also help to shed dead, hyperpigmented cells, causing a lightening effect by removing these dark dead cells. Use of a light-weight, non-comedogenic sunscreen on a daily basis will help prevent pigment caused by sun exposure. Comedogenic (clogged pore-causing) makeup and moisturizers must also be avoided.

It will take time to bring acne under control. If you have been using a routine anti-acne program for several weeks with no results, seek the advice of a qualified skin care professional or a dermatologist.

**Q** **I have some stiff, unwanted hairs on my chin. I try to keep them plucked, but I often get dark spots in the same area. What causes these dark spots?**

**A** These splotches in the area of unwanted hair are caused by ingrown hairs. Often, when hair is tweezed, the hair breaks inside the follicle below the skin surface and then grows into the follicle wall, causing inflammation and possible infection. The reaction is similar to that of an acne pimple forming.

Just like in a pimple, the inflammation causes stimulation of the melanocytes in the area, resulting in a dark spot forming. The treatment for this is the same as for acne pimples.

To avoid pigmenting in the area of superfluous hair, clip the hair close to the skin surface, rather than tweezing and possibly breaking the hair below the skin surface. You may want to consider electrolysis for these stiff hairs, which will permanently remove them.

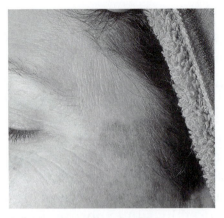

Solar lentigo, a "sun freckle".

 **What are "liver spots"?**

**A** Cumulative damage from sun overexposure over the years can cause overproduction of melanin in areas resulting in **solar lentigos,** commonly known as sun freckles, age spots, or "liver spots," which have nothing to do with the liver, other than the fact that they may be the same color as liver!

Solar lentigos commonly occur on the hands, arms, and face—areas that have been repeatedly exposed to sun without protection.

**Q** **What are the concepts in treating hyperpigmented skin?**

**A** The most important concept is to avoid sun and use a sunscreen on a daily basis. Ideally, this sunscreen should be built into a daily moisturizer that is individualized for the person's skin type. The sunscreen should be broad-spectrum and have an SPF of at least 15, although SPF 30+ is often recommended for skin with hyperpigmentation.

The second concept is to remove dead surface cells that are already stained with melanin, most often accomplished with the use of a chemical exfoliant, such as an alpha hydroxy acid (AHA). Glycolic acid and lactic acid are the most frequently used AHAs. The acid is usually in the form of a serum, gel, or lotion and may be used once or twice a day at home.

All AHA products must be used in conjunction with an SPF-15 or higher sunscreen, which is even more important when treating hyperpigmentation.

Alpha hydroxy acids work by dissolving the bond between dead cells, allowing surface cells to fall off the skin surface. Because these cells are already stained with pigment, removing them reveals cells underneath that may be non-stained, lighter in pigment content and color.

In many cases of minor splotchy mottling due to sun exposure, the use of an AHA gel or serum, along with sunscreen and sun avoidance, significantly lightens discolorations in a matter of weeks or months. Continued use of the products and sunscreen will result in further normalization of skin color.

The third concept in hyperpigmentation treatment is the use of a product that contains a melanin suppressant.

**Q** What is a melanin suppressant?

**A** A **melanin suppressant** is a topical substance that interferes with the biochemical process that produces melanin in skin cells. These agents work by chemically stopping physiological reactions that are needed for melanin to be formed in the skin.

The most commonly used melanin suppressant is a drug ingredient called **hydroquinone.** Hydroquinone is used in over-the-counter drug preparations in up to 2% concentration, and in prescription topical medications, hydroquinone is used in 4–6% concentrations, and occasionally higher. Hydroquinone is available in cream, lotion, gel, and serum forms.

Hydroquinone is often used in conjunction with keratolytic (peeling) and exfoliating agents such as alpha hydroxy acids or tretinoin (the active ingredient in Retin-A) or other retinoids. The exfoliating agents help with penetration of the hydroquinone, and removing surface keratinocytes (surface cells) that are already stained with melanin.

In prescription medications, hydroquinone may be combined with tretinoin and sometimes is combined with a steroid ingredient. This three-way combination is sometimes effective in treating stubborn melasma.

**Q** **Is there more than one type of melanin suppressant?**

**A** Hydroquinone is the only lightening drug agent approved for over-the-counter use, up to 2% concentration. Other performance agents, such as **arbutin, kojic acid,** and **bearberry extract,** are used in "skin brightening" products but are not, at this time, FDA-approved for over-the-counter use. All of these agents work in a similar manner to hydroquinone. Because these agents are not approved, it is unlawful to make claims of "lightening pigmentation," which is a drug claim that can only be made if using hydroquinone.

**Q** **Is topical vitamin C helpful in treating hyperpigmentation?**

**A** In mild cases, topical vitamin C can help lighten dark spots. In its ester form, **magnesium ascorbyl phosphate,** it is the most effective. It is used extensively throughout Asia in many skin care products. It is most effective when used with an alpha hydroxy acid serum and a good daily sunscreen.

**Q** **Are peels helpful in treating hyperpigmentation?**

**A** Mild alpha and beta hydroxy acid peels and other chemo-exfoliation treatments are used to remove hyperpigmented dead cell layers, making hyperpigmentation seem to fade. They can make a big difference in speeding up the fading of hyperpigmentation, but they must be performed carefully and accompanied by proper home care including a home AHA gel or serum, a good daily sunscreen, and a melanin suppressant.

**Q** **How often should AHA peels be performed for hyperpigmentation?**

**A** Most estheticians begin with six weekly or twice-weekly 30% pH 3.0 AHA treatments, preceded by home treatment with a 10% AHA serum or gel for at least 2 weeks prior to the first AHA peel. Biweekly peels may be used after the initial series if more lightening is desired. If the skin seems inflamed, flaky, or red, space the treatments further apart.

**Q** **Can aggressive peels make hyperpigmentation worse?**

**A** The type of AHA peels discussed above usually help hyperpigmentation and do not cause enough stimulation to worsen pigment problems.

Strong peels or too many peeling treatments are often overkill for many cases of hyperpigmentation, and the trauma caused by these peels can actually cause more pigment to form due to inflammation. This is particularly true in darker skin types. Similarly, microdermabrasion can remove hyperpigmented surface cells, but in some cases it can stimulate hyperpigmentation.

The trick in peeling hyperpigmented skin is to be gentle and conservative, to prepare the skin by using 10% alpha hydroxy acid exfoliating home care products for at least 2 weeks prior to any peeling treatment using AHA, and to use a sunscreen and melanin suppressant daily and avoid sun exposure. Be patient and wait to see how the skin responds to a short weekly or twice-weekly series of 30% AHA (pH 3.0) treatments by a well-trained skin care professional before proceeding to more aggressive treatment. Be aware that the more aggressive the peeling treatment, the more risk there is of worsening or flaring the hyper-pigmentation due to inflammation (PIH). More aggressive chemical treatment includes salicylic acid peels, Jessner's peels, and Unna peels (sulfur and resorcinol).

**Q** Are there medical treatments for hyperpigmentation?

**A** Yes. Dermatologists are the doctors that should be consulted for hyperpigmentation that does not respond to less-aggressive treatments. They have much more experience than many other types of physicians in treating complicated hyperpigmentation cases. They also are better acquainted with unique problems of hyperpigmentation in people of color.

The medical treatments generally are based on the same concepts already discussed, with the exception that physicians generally use more aggressive methods. For example, hydroquinone is available by prescription in strengths, usually 4–6%, much higher than the 2% available in over-the-counter preparations. Tretinoin (Retin-A) is often prescribed to accompany the hydroquinone. Another frequent prescription is Triluma, a combination of tretinoin, hydroquinone, and a steroid (fluocinolone acetonide), often used for treating melasma.

Stronger peels using TCA are performed in doctors' offices, as are many types of light therapies, such as intense pulsed light (IPL) treatments. Many types of lasers are also used to help clear hyperpigmentation as well. Lasers often do an efficient job removing pigmented cells, but if the hyperpigmentation is caused from hormone imbalances, this must also be addressed or the hyperpigmentation can return. Care must also be used to prevent hyperpigmentation that might be stimulated by the laser treatment. Often, the physician will prescribe hydroquinone to be used at home for a time before laser treatment.

**Q** Can I continue my salon peels while I am having medical treatment?

**A** Generally speaking, no. You should ask your dermatologist what types of cosmetic treatments are appropriate while you are under the dermatologist's care. Having a conditioning facial and using a good moisturizer is probably fine. But using additional peeling agents in addition to those prescribed by the dermatologist may cause too much exfoliation and possibly inflammation that may complicate the situation.

**Q** What about light spots that seem to be missing pigment? What causes these?

**A** Lack of pigment in the skin is called **hypopigmentation.** There are several causes for hypopigmentation:

- Sun damage or dermatoheliosis can cause absence of pigment from damage to the melanocytes. This is usually mixed in with splotchy hyperpigmentation, so it appears as a small area of light skin within a speckled area of various shades of hyperpigmentation. This occurs primarily in persons who have had excessive and frequent exposure to the sun.
- **Tinea versicolor** is a fungus that causes white spots on usually tanned skin. These light splotches are frequently seen on the backs and chests (and sometimes faces) of surfers and frequent beachgoers. The fungus inhibits the production of melanin in the areas that it is present.
- **Vitiligo** is a chronic condition, believed by some medical scientists to be an autoimmune disease, in which the skin loses the ability to make pigment. Vitiligo may also be genetic. The disease varies in effects. Some people have small areas of pigment loss, and others have widespread loss, to the point of an entire area of the body being a lighter color due to complete pigment loss.

It can be obvious in persons of color, and sometimes **depigmentation**—destroying pigment in the surrounding areas with the use of depigmenting drugs—may be used to even out the color.

Vitiligo has been associated with thyroid disease, but the majority of people with vitiligo have no other symptoms. There are some treatments for vitiligo, but none are 100% effective. The main treatment for re-pigmentation involves the use of a drug called **psoralen,** which is also used to treat psoriasis. Patients using psoralen are exposed to light boxes that stimulate melanin production. Again, this is rarely 100% effective.

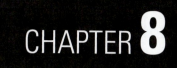

# CHAPTER 8

# Skin Care Products
# and Ingredients

151

**Q** **Why do some cleansers foam while others don't?**

**A** Foaming cleansers contain ingredients known as **surfactants.** Surfactants reduce the surface tension on the skin, allowing products to slip across the skin. Surfactants include **detergents** (*not* the concentration of laundry detergent!), commonly called cleansing agents. These ingredients remove oils, dirt, and sebum from the skin efficiently and also cause foam to form. The more a cleanser foams, the more surfactant it contains.

Cleansers that do not foam use oils or emollients to cleanse the skin. They are often called cleansing milks or cleansing creams. These are primarily used for makeup removal and for drier skin types.

**Q** **What are some surfactants commonly used for cleansing that I may see on an ingredient label?**

**A** The lauryl and laureth sulfates are the most common. Sodium lauryl sulfate is frequently used as the cleansing agent in shampoos and facial washes. Most people can use sodium lauryl sulfate without a problem, but it has been known to cause irritation and dryness in sensitive, redness-prone, dry, and acne-prone skin. It most likely causes irritation by stripping too much lipid (sebum) off the skin and affecting the lipids within the barrier function. Skin types with damaged barrier function, such as some of those listed above, may be more susceptible to further barrier damage and irritation. Ammonium lauryl sulfate is an alternative that is less irritating, although if it is in high concentration, it still may overclean the skin.

Cleansing agent surfactants are usually listed toward the beginning of the ingredient list, meaning that they are in high concentration. Ingredients are listed on an ingredient label in order of their concentration in the product. So, the ingredients that make up the majority of the product are listed first, and the ingredients that are used in small quantities are listed at the end of the list.

Other common cleansing agents include cocamidopropyl betaine, disodium lauryl sulfosuccinate, and decyl polyglucoside.

**Q** **How do I choose the best cleanser for my skin?**

**A** The oilier your skin is, the more you need to use a foaming surfactant-type cleanser. Foaming cleansers do a better job of removing excess oils. The best choice of foaming cleanser will depend on the degree of oiliness of your skin. The strength of a foaming cleanser is determined by the amount of surfactant it contains. Acne-prone skin may need a medicated cleanser with benzoyl peroxide or salicylic acid. Very oily skin might need a cleanser that foams a lot, while a combination skin might need a cleanser that only foams a small amount.

Dry and sensitive skin should use cleansing products with little or no detergent. They should foam little, if at all. It is important that cleansers for dry or sensitive skin do not remove too much sebum. The sebum on the surface of these skin types helps to protect the fragile barrier function that, when stripped, allows the cleanser to begin to eat away at the barrier function. Continual use of such a product may result in dryness, flaking, redness, and irritation.

Generally speaking, dry and sensitive skin should use cleansing milks that do not foam or foam very little. Decyl glucoside is a gentle cleansing agent that is suitable for many people with dry and sensitive skin. It allows for a small amount of foaming, which can make a product easier to rinse off and also more convenient to use. Products for these skin types should also be fragrance-free and contain no stimulants. They may also contain emollient or lipid agents to buffer the contact of the surfactants with the skin, or may contain special soothing or conditioning ingredients to avoid drying from cleansing and to soothe any irritation caused during the cleansing process.

Nonfoaming cleansing milks are best to use for makeup removal for all skin types. Makeup is cleansed from the skin much more effectively with an emollient, nonfoaming cleanser. These cleansing milks should be used with a damp, soft cleansing cloth or cotton pads to help remove makeup and other debris from the skin.

If you have combination skin, as many people do, you should use a foaming cleanser appropriate for your oiliness level in the morning in the shower, and use a cleansing milk at night to remove makeup.

**Q** **Should I use cold or hot water to clean my skin? Doesn't hot water kill bacteria and open pores?**

**A** Everyone should use room temperature water on his or her skin at all times. Hot water irritates skin and dilates blood vessels and is terrible for sensitive skin and rosacea. Hot water does not get hot enough to kill bacteria without burning the skin. If you have acne, a medicated cleanser will work to kill bacteria without using hot water.

Pores do not open and close like gates. Water is the magic, not the heat. Pre-wetting the skin before applying a cleanser will help do a better job loosening sebum and debris.

Cold water is unpleasant and can also cause issues for skin with rosacea.

**Q** **Should I use a cleansing cloth or sponge when I clean my face?**

**A** It is a good idea to use a cleansing cloth or facial sponge when cleansing your skin, especially during makeup removal. For cleansing milks, damp cotton pads are also great—they are gentle and disposable. They are also perfect for the delicate skin around the eyes.

Avoid using any rough implement on the skin when cleansing. Rough washcloths and scratchy pads can cause micro-abrasions on the skin.

Cleansing implements should be used only once before washing the implement or sanitizing it.

**Q** **I don't feel clean unless I have washed my face. Is it okay to wash my face after I remove the makeup with a cleansing milk?**

**A** Yes, after carefully removing your makeup, it is fine to wash your face as long as the wash (foaming cleanser) is appropriate for your oiliness level.

**Q** **What do toners do? Do I really need a toner?**

**A** Toners have several important functions.

- Cleansers often raise the pH on the skin during the cleansing process, making it more alkaline. Toners restore the slightly acid level of the skin surface by lowering the pH after cleansing. The ideal pH for the skin surface is between 5.5 and 6.2.
- Toners sometimes contain defatting agents that clean up cleanser or makeup residue that might be left on the face. This is particularly true of those toners designed for oilier skin.
- Toners help to refine the appearance of the pores by making them look smaller. Toners may also contain agents that temporarily tighten the skin surface.
- Toners often contain hydrating agents that help to attract water to the skin surface before a moisturizer is applied.
- Toners can contain soothing agents that help to calm redness after cleansing. Toners are an important part of a complete skin care program. It is important to choose the right one for your skin type.

**Q** **What ingredients should I look for in a good moisturizer?**

**A** Moisturizers are mixtures of **emollients** to keep moisture in the skin and hydrators or humectants to attract water to the skin. All moisturizers are mixtures of these two ingredient types. They vary by the content of each, and by other ingredients that may be in the formulation.

Which ingredients to look for and how much of each one to use depends on your skin type. If you have oily or combination skin, you probably already make enough sebum, which serves as a natural emollient to keep moisture in the skin. This means that you need more humectant and less emollient. Your skin might feel dry because it might be dehydrated. You need water, not oil!

If your skin has few or no visible pores, you have skin that is not making enough sebum, which serves as a natural emollient. Your skin can also become dehydrated, but the fact that you do not make enough natural emollient is a major factor, unlike combination or oily skin. You need a moisturizer that has added emollient, often oils or a lipid component to hold water in the skin.

Frequently used humectant ingredients include sodium hyaluronate, glycerin, sorbitol, butylene glycol, and sodium PCA. Emollients are numerous including many natural oils such as jojoba, avocado, and sunflower oils; fats such as capric/caprylic triglycerides; and fatty acids and esters, as well as waxes. Silicones and derivatives such as cyclopentasiloxane serve as both spreading agents and moisture-guarding protectants.

**Q** **Why are some moisturizers creams and some lotions?**

**A** Moisturizing creams generally have more emollient content and therefore have a thicker consistency. They are generally designed for dry skin lacking sebum, so if you have dry skin with small or barely visible pores, this type of product might be a good choice for your skin. Creams also may have more emulsifier to thoroughly mix the water and oils or emollients in the formulation. They are normally sold in jars or tubes. Lotions have a higher water content than creams and are generally designed for oilier or combination skin types.

**Q** My dermatologist recommended a moisturizing lotion that contains petrolatum. Isn't petrolatum clogging to the skin?

**A** No. Fatty esters, which are smaller fatty molecules, are much more likely to cause comedones (clogged pores) to develop. Petrolatum in its pure form (petroleum jelly) is obviously greasy, hence its erroneous reputation as a pore-clogging ingredient. When blended into an emulsion (cream or lotion), this greasiness seems to disappear. Petrolatum is probably the best emollient ingredient for preventing moisture loss. It is **biologically inert,** which means it does not cross-react with chemicals in the body, making it great to use for reactive or allergy-prone, sensitive skin.

Unfortunately, petrolatum is used less and less in formulations due to its ill-rumored reputation. It is an excellent ingredient for treating dry skin, especially dry body skin.

**Q** My moisturizer has cetyl alcohol in it. Isn't alcohol drying to the skin?

**A** Not all alcohols are drying. When most people think of alcohol, they think of isopropyl (rubbing) alcohol, which is drying and stings when it comes in contact with a scratch or abrasion on the skin. SD alcohol is another cosmetic alcohol that has a drying effect.

*Alcohol* is a chemical term that simply means that a hydrogen atom and an oxygen atom have attached themselves to the end of a carbon chain. Most alcohols are actually fatty based, which means they are more like a creamy emollient or might even have a waxy texture. They are primarily used as emollients in moisturizers or other cream or lotion formulations. Cetyl alcohol is both an emollient and an emulsifier, keeping creams or lotions uniformly mixed.

**Q** **Is there any real difference between a moisturizer and an eye cream?**

**A** Yes. The skin around the eye is much thinner, more delicate, and more sensitive than other facial areas. It is has fewer sebaceous glands and is probably the most fragile skin on the entire body, and most likely to show signs of premature aging and sun damage.

Modern eye creams are carefully formulated to treat this delicate tissue. Eye creams generally contain more emollient or lipids than general moisturizers to compensate for the lack of sebum in this area. They may also contain some state-of-the-art ingredients such as peptides (see below), enzymes, lipids, and antioxidants, which help to improve appearance problems such as puffiness, dark circles, fine lines and wrinkles, and dry texture.

**Q** **What are peptides?**

**A** Technically, peptides are chains of amino acids, the most basic building block of proteins. When amino acids are joined they are peptides. When peptides are joined they are proteins.

In modern skin care science, peptides are used to prompt the skin to behave in a particular way, changing the appearance of some part of the skin. Groups of amino acids are combined to form peptides, which are combined with a fatty component to more easily penetrate the skin.

The best-known peptide in skin care science is palmitoyl pentapeptide-3, also known as Matrixyl. It is used in anti-aging formulations to help improve texture and elasticity of the skin.

The sequence of amino acids in this peptide is the same as they are in a piece of a collagen molecule. By introducing this peptide to the skin, it is theorized that it "tricks" the skin into "believing" that the collagen is already broken down, causing the skin to respond biochemically by slowing collagen-breakdown enzymes. This results in a firmer look to the skin and lessening in the appearance of lines and wrinkles.

**Q** **Is there more than one kind of peptide?**

**A** There are many, many types of peptides. Research is ongoing as to which may influence the appearance of the skin. Some make a difference and some do not.

Some other forms of peptides currently used in skin care include **palmitoyl oligopeptide** and **palmitoyl tetrapeptide,** used together for firming and to improve wrinkle appearance; **dipeptide-2,** used for eye puffiness; and **acetyl hexapeptide-8,** used to relax the appearance of wrinkles, primarily in the facial expressions.

Peptide products can be combined with other different performance agents or products to produce even more effective results.

**Q** **What do exfoliators do?**

**A** Exfoliators remove dead cells from the skin surface, revealing a smoother surface, helping to make wrinkles and lines look less deep, and generally helping facial texture. By clearing the skin surface of the excess dead cells, they enable products to work more efficaciously by allowing better absorption and delivery of any treatment product. If used correctly, they stimulate cell renewal, improving hydration. If overused, they can cause irritation and dryness.

**Q** **Is there more than one type of exfoliant?**

**A** There are two basic kinds of exfoliators:

■ Mechanical exfoliators include facial scrubs, cleansing beads, exfoliating masks, and roll-off (gommage) products. They work by physically removing dead cells from the skin surface. Sometimes they are mixed into a cleanser for easy use. Microdermabrasion is another form of mechanical exfoliation.

- Chemical exfoliants work by chemically dissolving the dead cells or the bonds between the dead cells on the skin surface. Chemical exfoliants, unlike mechanical exfoliators, can penetrate follicles, helping with follicular debris such as comedones, enlarged pores, and breakout problems. Chemical exfoliators are primarily acids or enzymes. Acids include beta hydroxy salicylic acid and alpha hydroxy glycolic, malic, mandelic, and other acids. Sulfur can also be used as a chemical exfoliant, as can benzoyl peroxide. Enzymes include papain (from papaya) and bromelain (from pineapple). They are proteolytic (protein-dissolving) enzymes that dissolve the keratin in the dead surface keratinocytes.

Both mechanical and chemical exfoliators are available in at-home strengths for consumer use, as well as much stronger versions for professional use by estheticians or in dermatology.

**Q** What are the benefits of using an alpha hydroxy acid treatment product?

**A** Alpha hydroxy acids are probably the most effective and versatile performance ingredients in skin care science today. They work by dissolving the bond between surface corneocytes, promoting a variety of skin care improvements:

- Smoothing the skin surface and texture—by removing pile-ups of dead cells, alpha hydroxy acids even out the skin surface, improving smoothness and texture. They remove "pile-ups" on the sides of wrinkles and lines, softening their appearance and improving the way light reflects off the skin, making skin look much smoother.
- Alpha hydroxy acids help to flush debris from follicles, loosening comedones and debris to be expelled from the follicles, therefore improving the appearance of

pores and also helping prevent impactions that can lead to acne lesions.

- Alpha hydroxy acids remove melanin-infused keratinocytes making skin color appear more even looking and reducing the appearance of dark splotches and hyperpigmented areas.
- By removing dead cells from the skin surface, alpha hydroxy acids promote cell renewal. It is the cell renewal process that causes the corneum to form the important lipids that form the barrier function of the skin. Therefore, use of alpha hydroxy acids improves the moisture binding capabilities of the epidermis. This, in turn, also makes skin look smoother and firmer by increasing hydration of the skin.

**Q** **What should I look for in an alpha hydroxy acid home care treatment product?**

**A** First, to see any real improvement in the skin's appearance, alpha hydroxy acid products must be used routinely. Some cleansers contain alpha hydroxy acids. These should not be considered treatment products. AHAs used in cleansers are in the product to improve efficacy, but these products do not stay on the skin long enough to instill any change.

Alpha hydroxy home care treatment products are available in lotion, serum, gel, and cream forms. They must be *worn* for hours at a time to be effective. You should choose the product form that best suits your skin type.

A good AHA product will contain 8–10% alpha hydroxy acid, which often is a mix of glycolic and lactic acids. It may contain additional acids, including beta hydroxy salicylic acid.

Some alpha hydroxy acid products in lotion and cream forms can also serve as moisturizers.

Home-care AHA products should have a pH no lower than 3.5. Products with pHs lower than 3.5 will have a tendency to produce irritation and inflammation.

**Q.** **Are there any precautions for using alpha hydroxy acid products?**

**A** Alpha hydroxy acids can be effective for many skin problems, but there are a number of precautions you should take or be aware of prior to using such a product:

- Alpha hydroxy acid products work by exfoliating the skin and should not be used at the same time as other exfoliating products, including prescription exfoliators such as Retin-A, Differin, or Tazorac, unless under the direction of a dermatologist. To use more than one exfoliant concurrently can cause inflammation, peeling, and reactivity to other products. AHAs should not be used during or for several months after taking Accutane (isotretinoin). Check with your dermatologist about when it might be appropriate to resume using an AHA product. Likewise, one should not use harsh mechanical exfoliants with AHA products. Any mechanical exfoliant used while using AHA products should be administered carefully.
- Use the product according to manufacturer's directions.
- If you have sensitive skin, you should be careful choosing an AHA product. Sensitive skin can usually use AHAs, but you need to be careful with concentration and pH factors. It is a good idea to consult a qualified skin care professional. Secondly, some people with sensitive skin may need to use AHA products less often than persons with nonsensitive skin.
- Be careful if waxing areas of skin where AHAs have been used. AHAs can thin the surface of the skin, making some individuals more susceptible to side effects of waxing such as excessive irritation and even possible accidental peeling of the skin in the treated area. If you are using AHAs or any other topical exfoliant, make sure you go to a qualified skin care therapist for waxing services, and make sure they are aware you are using a topical exfoliant before your waxing treatment.

- Using alpha hydroxy acids may make persons more susceptible to sunburn. While using an AHA product, you must always use a broad-spectrum SPF-15 or higher sunscreen (as you should anyway at all times!).
- If having a professional alpha hydroxy acid exfoliation treatment by an esthetician or dermatologist, you should use an 8–10% concentration home care product on a daily basis for at least 2 weeks prior to having the professional exfoliation treatment. Skin that has not been prepared with pretreatment at home will be much more likely to have irritant reactions.

It is best to use alpha hydroxy acids under the direction of a skin care professional. They have lots of experience in using these products and can give you good advice on their safe and effective use. They can also advise you about professional higher concentration exfoliation treatments. Also known as AHA peels, these treatments can boost your program when performed in a series.

**Q** What are liposomes? How do they work?

**A** **Liposomes** are tiny encapsulation vessels that are often filled with performance skin care ingredients. Liposomes are made of a fatty substance, often soy lecithin or phospholipids. Because they are made of lipids, they are more easily accepted by the lipids between cells, which allow them to penetrate the skin surface.

When the liposome penetrates into the lipid matrix between the cells, the liposome shell becomes a part of the matrix, releasing the performance ingredient.

Liposomes are important because they transport ingredients to where they are needed, and because they protect ingredients such as antioxidants from being used or oxidized before they reach their destination in the skin.

Not all ingredients can or should be microencapsulated. Some ingredient complexes are simply too big to put in a liposome. Some ingredients, such as sunscreen, need to stay on the skin surface to work best.

**Q** **What are antioxidants and why are they so important for the skin?**

**A** **Antioxidants** are natural substances that occur in the body as well as in nature. Antioxidants prevent or squelch oxidation, which is the process of natural biochemicals losing electrons to **oxidizers,** which are chemicals, often oxygen-based, that steal electrons from the biochemicals, causing inflammation and interfering with normal cellular functioning. These wild oxygen components are commonly known as free radicals.

Oxidation is a normal biological process, but when there is too much oxidation in the body or the skin, a series of biochemical reactions occur that eventually results in damage to cells, tissues, and skin. Allowing these reactions to go unchecked will result in skin damage appearing as wrinkles, sagging, and other signs of aging.

Antioxidants work in and on the skin by stopping these cascades of biochemical reactions that lead to skin damage that creates the appearance effects of aging skin. They either neutralize free radicals or block these inflammatory reactions.

Antioxidants are present in colorful fruits and vegetables, which are the best natural source for them. Topical and supplemental antioxidants are also frequently used and advised.

Antioxidants frequently used in skin care include concentrated forms of plant extracts such as green tea, grapeseed, licorice, and pomegranate. There are many different antioxidants that can be used in skin care products.

**Q** **Are topical vitamins effective for the skin? How do they help?**

**A** There is no question that certain vitamins can improve the appearance and condition of the skin. Most scientists believe that vitamins work because they are antioxidants, protecting the skin against oxidative damage that can cause inflammation and eventual damage leading to what we see as aging of the skin.

The most popular vitamin ingredients used in skin care products are the following:

- Vitamin A—also known as **retinol**—has many effects on the skin including antioxidant activity. Retinol is frequently used in anti-aging products because it is necessary for normal cell growth and function, and it helps to modulate collagen synthesis. This results in more youthful-looking skin. Vitamin A derivatives are known as **retinoids** and include topical skin drugs such as Retin-A, Tazorac, and Differin, as well as the oral acne drug Accutane (isotretinoin). There are also other skin care ingredients derived from vitamin A, such as retinyl aldehyde and retinyl palmitate.

- Vitamin C is also known as **l-ascorbic acid** and is used in skin care products as magnesium ascorbyl phosphate, **sodium ascorbyl phosphate,** and **ascorbyl palmitate.** Primarily used for treatment of aging and sun-damaged skin, these strong antioxidants help prevent damage to cell membranes from oxidation, and vitamin C is also necessary for collagen production. Vitamin C is also effective as a skin brightener, helping to even out uneven skin pigment and mottling caused from sun damage.

- Vitamin E, known in skin care products as **tocopherol** or **tocopheryl acetate,** is a fat-soluble vitamin that serves as an antioxidant for the skin, as well as a preservative antioxidant for the products themselves. It is particularly effective when used in conjunction with vitamin C.

- **Panthenol,** also known as vitamin B5, has long been used as a moisturizing ingredient in moisturizers. Panthenol is also necessary for normal cell functioning.

- **Ergocalciferol,** also known as vitamin D, is a fat-soluble vitamin. Vitamin D is quickly gaining attention and is now believed by many scientists to be much more important to the body in general than once thought. Vitamin D is involved in the skin in cell renewal and may have many more functions.

These are only a few vitamins that are used topically. There are many more vitamins as well as minerals used in skin care.

**Q** **Are there certain things I should look for in a good antioxidant product?**

**A** There can be big differences in antioxidant treatment products. Simply adding some antioxidant to a moisturizer does not necessarily mean it will help your skin.

The best antioxidant products are often in serum form. The base (spreading agent) of these products makes the serum penetrate better than if they were mixed into a moisturizer.

It is important to look for a product that has several different antioxidants in it. There are many types of free radicals. They are sometimes called **reactive oxygen species (ROS).** The different types of free radicals are squelched by different kinds of antioxidants. A **broad-spectrum antioxidant** serum contains numerous antioxidants to squelch a variety of oxidative reactions.

Antioxidant ingredients should be protected so that they do not work before they are applied to the skin. Antioxidants that are not protected will oxidize in the package and often turn dark or brown.

Using liposomes or other encapsulation methods helps to protect the antioxidant ingredients and also helps the ingredients to penetrate the skin surface easier. Vitamin E or tocopherol, for example, will work as an antioxidant in the product instead of on the skin unless it is protected.

Finally, look for a product that is comfortable and easy to use. Antioxidant serums are typically applied before moisturizers or sunscreens. The product should not sting or cause redness. Make sure that you enjoy the feel of the product because it will not work if it is not used!

**Q** **Are there ingredients to treat redness?**

**A** Ingredients that claim to reduce inflammation are technically drugs. The only over-the-counter drug ingredient that can make this drug claim is hydrocortisone. However, there are cosmetic ingredients that have a soothing and calming effect on the skin, reducing the appearance of redness or helping to prevent problems that can bring out redness.

Color cosmetics with green bases are promoted to neutralize redness, but these products are strictly cosmetic. They do not calm the skin. They simply cover up and disguise the redness.

Many of the antioxidants mentioned earlier are calming to the skin, probably because they inhibit the free radicals that can lead to inflammation. **Grapeseed** and **green tea extracts** and **matricaria** (from chamomile) **extract** are frequently used in calming products. **Lichochalcone,** derived from licorice, is a strong antioxidant used in products to curb irritancy. **Dipotassium glycyrrhizinate,** also derived from licorice, and **elizabethae extract,** from a coral called **sea whip,** are both excellent calmers.

There are many ingredients that might be avoided in sensitive skin or rosacea that might cause irritation in redness-prone skin. These include fragrances, many essential oils, drying alcohols, and other stimulating ingredients. For much more information on this subject, see the chapter on sensitive skin.

**Q** **Why are preservatives used in skin care and cosmetic products?**

**A** Preservatives are extremely important ingredients in the development of skin care products. They protect the products from pathogenic contamination and also help to keep creams and products fresh. Without them, skin care products would spoil and grow microbial cultures quickly! Preservatives kill bacteria that can harm the skin, eyes, or body, and the preservatives also help protect against cross-contamination from things such as fingers in the jar.

Any product that contains water can support microbial life. Likewise, any product containing naturally derived ingredients can sustain microbes.

Products that claim to be preservative-free generally contain no water or natural ingredients, or they must be used quickly. Petrolatum in its pure state, for example, does not need a preservative. It contains no water and comes from minerals instead of being biologically derived.

**Q** **How important is it to buy "natural" skin care?**

**A** There are many great things that come from nature, and many cosmetic and skin care ingredients are derived from plants. Up to 1/3 of all chemicals used in prescription drugs are also plant-derived.

Many people erroneously believe that products made from natural substances are safer or are free of chemicals. The truth is that all things are made from chemicals! Plant extracts are simply complexes of many chemicals produced by nature. When pure chemicals are produced in the laboratory, they are often isolated from natural sources.

There are plenty of natural things that are not safe. Poison ivy is only one of many plants that contain harmful natural chemicals. Coconut oil and cocoa butter can cause clogged pores in acne patients. "Natural" might mean derived from nature, but is does not necessarily mean chemical-free, safe, or effective. Likewise, synthetic or laboratory-produced does not mean that the ingredient is toxic or bad for the body. It is the opinion of this author that we should use the best of all worlds in creating great skin care products. There are effective and useful ingredients that come from both nature and the laboratory.

**Q** **Are there any bad ingredients that everyone should avoid?**

**A** If there were such bad ingredients, they would be taken off the market by the FDA.

There are no bad ingredients, just bad applications of use for certain ingredients. For example, there are fatty acids and oils such as coconut oil that can wreak havoc and clog up acne and clog-prone skin. These same fats may help an oil-dry skin. People often enjoy fragrances, but fragrances can be definite irritants for sensitive skin; SD alcohol may help control excess sebum for oily skin but can dry and irritate a dry, sensitive skin.

If you have sensitive, acne-prone, or dry skin, there are certain ingredients you should avoid. Much of this is common sense, but everyone with skin problems should consult with a skin care professional or dermatologist about which ingredients they should avoid and which might help their skin.

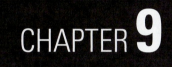

CHAPTER **9**

# Your Personal Skin Analysis

**Q** How can I tell if I have oily, dry, or combination skin?

**A** When a skin care professional looks at someone's facial skin, the first thing he or she observes is the distribution of pores on the face. Carefully examining the size and location of obvious pore openings, he or she can determine the following:

- Skin with large visible pores all across the skin, including the skin near the ears, is **oily skin.** The larger pores are due to the follicles being expanded to accommodate the large amount of sebum flowing through them. Oily skin sometimes is said to have "orange peel texture." It is often shiny and may have a waxy texture. It often has clogged pores and may have open comedones (blackheads) or closed comedones (small bumps just under the skin).

- If it is hard to see the pores, even with a magnifying lamp, the skin is likely dry or alipidic. The pores are not easily visible to the eye because they are not dilated much due to lack of sebum, which normally flows through the follicle, stretching the follicle and therefore the opening the pore. Skin that does not produce enough sebum often also will have a non-smooth feeling to the touch, like fine sandpaper. It is often dehydrated from lack of protection, may have many small wrinkles, and may be slightly flaky.

- If the skin has visible pores down the middle of the face, and the pores start becoming smaller as your focus moves toward the perimeter of the face (toward the ears), this is **combination skin.** Like its name, it is a mix of oily and dry areas. Most often the oily area is down the center of the face, and the dry areas with smaller pores are around the edges (perimeter) of the face. Combination skin may have both symptoms of oily skin in the oily areas and symptoms of dry skin in the drier areas.

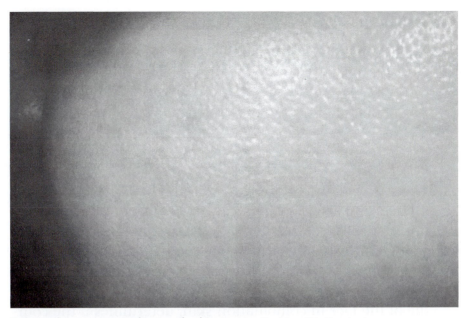

Enlarged pore areas indicate oily skin *(courtesy Mark Lees Skin Care, Inc.)*.

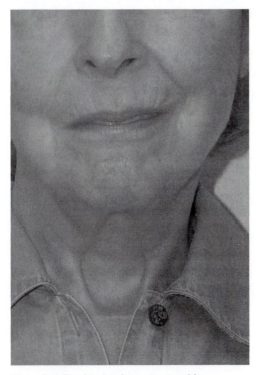

Dry, alipidic skin is characterized by
non-visible pores *(courtesy Mark Lees Skin Care, Inc.)*.

**Q** **Why do people have different skin types?**

**A** Skin types are determined by genetics. You inherit your skin type. Oiliness and dryness can be affected by hormones and hormone fluctuations, disease, drugs (both prescription and recreational), and sometimes environment.

**Q** **Are there varying degrees of oiliness or dryness in individuals?**

**A** There are many differences in individuals. The degree of oiliness and dryness can be affected by genetics, hormones, and environment, including how the skin is cared for. Skin that is neglected, regardless of type, will have many more symptoms of conditions associated with that skin type.

   The width of the **T-zone,** the oily area down the middle of the face in combination skin, determines if the combination skin is oilier or drier. If the pores in the T-zone are easily visible and expand across the cheeks to an imaginary line from the corners of the eyes down, the skin is known as combination-oily. If the pores in the T-zone are visible in a narrow area down the center of the face, the skin is combination-dry. Most people have combination skin.

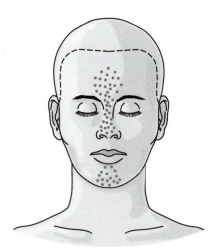

Typical distribution of oily and dry areas in the T-zone.

Because of genetics and hormones, most people produce less sebum as they get older and hence have drier skin when they are older.

**Q** What is "normal skin"?

**A** The truth is that few people have "normal skin," which is defined as having perfectly even sebum and pore distribution, not likely to be reactive or allergy-prone, and unlikely to have conditions of oiliness or dryness.

**Q** If I have combination skin, do I treat it as oily or dry?

**A** Most skin care products on the market are designed for combination skin and termed for "normal skin." Because most people have combination skin, it is accepted by marketers that combination skin is "normal."

You should choose products that lean toward your predominant skin type. Most skin care companies will clearly state on the label for what type of skin the product is intended. If you have questions, you should consult a skin care professional.

**Q** I am oily by 11 a.m. Does that mean I have oily skin?

**A** It is likely that you have oily skin, especially if you experience this when you are not wearing any makeup or moisturizer.

Oily makeup or an oily moisturizer could possibly make your oiliness increase with activity. If you are not experiencing oiliness at other times, your choice of makeup or moisturizer might be the problem.

Try switching to a lighter weight moisturizer or a powder mineral makeup. There are liquid foundations with evaporating bases designed for especially oily skin. Switching to this type of makeup should help with the morning oiliness.

There are also oil-absorbing products that contain silica or nylon to help absorb excess sebum on the skin surface. They are marketed as anti-shine products.

**Q** **Do I really need a moisturizer if I have oily skin?**

**A** You do not need an emollient moisturizer, but you still need some protection during the day, and definitely sunscreen!

Look for a lightweight sunscreen designed for oily skin that contains dimethicone or cyclopentasiloxane (both silicone derivatives), which will help your skin retain moisture and avoid surface dehydration without making your skin oilier.

Not every oily skin needs a night moisturizer. Look for a water-based serum with great ingredients such as anti-oxidants or peptides.

**Q** **I seem to have oily skin, but the surface seems really dry. Is it possible to have oily and dry skin in the same area?**

**A** If you have larger visible pores, and you are aware of the oiliness of your skin, you have oily skin. The "dryness" that you feel is probably dehydration, which is a condition, not a skin type. You have oily, dehydrated skin. The surface of your skin has a lack of water rather than a lack of oil. Dehydration is what causes skin to be flaky, tight, sometimes itchy or red, or have a cellophane-like appearance.

Dehydration in oily skin is often caused by overcleaning the skin, using harsh soaps, not using any moisturizer, or sun exposure.

**Q** **How do you treat dehydrated, oily skin?**

**A** Stop using harsh soap and alcohol-based products. Switch to a mild foaming cleanser with a cleansing agent such as ammonium lauryl sulfate. This should rinse easily and thoroughly. A mild toner, preferably with no alcohol or fragrance, should be used after cleansing.

Look for a moisturizer and sunscreen that is lightweight in texture and designed for oily-combination skin. With oily skin, you should always check to make sure the product has tested non-comedogenic, so it will not clog pores.

Remember, when treating dehydrated, oily skin, the skin needs water-binder or humectant, not emollients. The skin is making enough of its own protective emollient in the form of sebum. Oilier moisturizers are just going to make the skin oilier.

Look for moisturizers, sunscreens, or treatment products that contain hydrating agents such as sodium PCA, glycerin, or sodium hyaluronate. These ingredients will help to attract water to the skin without increasing the oiliness.

**Q** **What are those little bumps I get in my blush line?**

**A** They are most likely closed comedones, a type of pore impaction just under the skin surface likely caused by some of the ingredients in your blush. Certain types of D & C red dyes, which are coal tar derivatives, are comedogenic, which means they cause comedones to form.

Pressing agents, used to form powder blush into a cake in a compact, are usually some sort of waxy agent. These, too, may be comedogenic.

Not everyone is affected by this phenomenon. You must have a hereditary tendency to form comedones or develop acne to have this clogging problem.

**Q** **What can I do to clear these blush line bumps?**

**A** Stop using your current makeup on that area. The most likely culprit is your blush, but it could be your foundation or powder.

Look for products that claim that they are tested for comedogenicity. These products will normally contain carmine or iron oxides as colorants rather than D & C red dyes. Also, powder blush should be pressed with a non-comedogenic pressing agent such as zinc stearate, octyldodecyl steroyl stearate, or a silicone derivative such as cyclomethicone. Pressing agents such as isopropyl myristate or palmitate, lanolin or lanolates are more likely to be comedogenic.

Daily use of an alpha/beta hydroxy gel or 2.5% benzoyl peroxide gel will help clear these bumps from your skin. Professional extraction by a licensed skin care professional will help to quickly clear these comedones. Ask your skin care professional to recommend products that will help you clear this area and makeup products that will avoid these bumps recurring.

**Q** **I break out easily. Does that mean I have sensitive skin?**

**A** It depends on the type of breakout reaction. If you break out in a rash, hives, or red splotches easily or frequently or if your skin is itching or stinging, you probably have sensitive, allergy-prone skin, or maybe rosacea if it is on the face. This is particularly true if you are able to correlate the use of a product or an activity with your flares of inflammation. You should seek the help of a dermatologist who may be able to properly diagnose the problem. Skin care specialists can help you select products that may be appropriate for your sensitive skin.

If you break out in acne pimples, this does not mean your skin is sensitive. It means your skin is acne-prone and has a hereditary tendency to develop clogged pores and acne-type pimples.

You should be using a daily follicle exfoliant such as alpha/beta hydroxy acid gel or benzoyl peroxide to flush debris from the follicles. You should also make sure you are using a good cleanser that removes excess oil from the skin, and that all of your makeup and skin care products are designed for acne-prone skin and are non-comedogenic. If you need help, you should consult a skin care professional who specializes in problem skin treatment.

**Q** My skin develops clogs easily, but I am 40 and worried about aging. I try a lot of antiaging products, but they seem to make my clogged pores worse. Is there a solution for this?

**A** Because many people with aging skin also have dry skin, many treatment products designed to treat aging skin are also emollient-infused to supplement the lack of sebum in these dry skin types.

Your skin already makes more than enough sebum. This is why your skin is oily and you tend to develop clogged pores easily. The emollients in these dry skin products add fats to your already oily skin. This is why your clogged pores and breakouts seem to get worse when you use these products.

It is possible to find products that address both aging and clog-prone or acne-prone skin. Performance ingredients for aging skin management such as peptides, alpha hydroxy acids, sunscreen actives, and antioxidants are not comedogenic or the problem. The problem is the vehicle or spreading agent of the product, which often consist of fatty emollient ingredients, which will help dry, alipidic skin but will clog oily and acne-prone skin.

Look for products that contain the aforementioned performance ingredients, yet are lightweight and in fluid, gel, serum, or liquid form, rather than emollient-laden creams that feel heavier or oily when applied to the skin. Most products that are intended for breakout-prone or clog-prone skin are promoted for this skin type, and you will see them on the label. Look for claims of "independent-tested for comedogenicity" or non-comedogenic on the label.

If you have trouble finding products that meet your needs, consult a skin care professional.

**Q** I have bad bags under my eyes. What can help these?

**A** Bags under the eyes are caused by fluid retention and/or fat deposits in the lower lid area. Fat deposits under the eyes are generally hereditary. Because the skin is thin through this area, the fat causes a bulging effect.

This area retains fluids easily, resulting in puffiness. Persons who suffer from sinus congestion have even more of a problem with puffiness. Some drugs have a side effect of causing both eye as well as facial puffiness.

Morning puffiness is common and generally subsides after the person is awake and moving around. Facial massage, moving the facial muscles, and allowing the face to stay under the flow of a body temperature shower may help expedite reduction of the puffiness.

There are several skin care product types that help to reduce eye area puffiness:

- Compress solutions made of soothing or mildly astringent ingredients such as black tea or cucumber extract are used to soak cotton pads, which are applied to the eyes, with the head in an elevated position. This will quickly minimize puffiness due to congestion.
- Film-forming gels designed to tighten the eye-area skin when applied physically pull up on the tissue, reducing the look of puffiness. This is temporary, and when the product is removed, the skin is no longer tight.

One of the newer types of products features a peptide, known as dipeptide-2, along with a bioflavanoid called hesperidin methyl chalcone. The peptide helps strengthen capillaries to avoid fluid leakage, and the hesperedin methyl chalcone helps to reduce fluid. This more modern combination of ingredients has a longer-range treatment effect in terms of puffiness reduction. None of these products does anything to remove the fat pad in the lower lid.

**Q** Is there a more permanent solution for eye bags?

**A** Surgical removal of the fat pad or herniation under the eyes is the only permanent solution. This surgery is known as lower lid **blepharoplasty.** It is performed by facial plastic surgeons, ophthalmic plastic surgeons, or general plastic surgeons. The procedure is usually performed on an outpatient basis, and recovery is only a few days. Most people only need the procedure performed once, as recurrence of the fat pads is unlikely.

**Q** **I don't have bags under my eyes, but I have problems with dark circles. What causes these?**

**A** Darkness under the eyes is a problem for many and can be caused by a number of factors:

- The actual genetic structure of the bones around the eyes can make eyes look darker. Deep-set eyes will have a darker look due to shadowing and bone structure.
- Darkness under the eyes can also be caused by hyperpigmentation. This is prevalent in persons of Middle Eastern descent.
- Most darkness under the eyes is caused by poor blood circulation and leakage of blood cells that get "stuck" in the tissues around the eyes. The hemoglobin from these red blood cells, and pigments caused from degraded hemoglobin, cause a dark appearance.
- Lack of sleep and stress also seem to increase eye circle darkness, probably due to poorer circulation during these times of stress. In some people sinus swelling can also result in a worse appearance of dark circles.

**Q** **How can I tell if my circles are due to hyperpigmentation or blood circulation?**

**A** Gently pull the lower lid skin outwards or press on the circle area. If the skin color gets lighter, the problem is circulatory. If the skin stays dark, the problem is hyperpigmentation. The action of pushing on the skin tissue causes blood to move away, lightening the appearance of the area.

**Q** How can you treat the different types of eye circle darkness?

**A** Eye circles caused by pigmentation can be treated with a kojic acid eye cream or a mild hydroquinone product. Make sure you choose one designed for eye areas, and patch test it on a small area to make sure it does not cause an allergic or irritant reaction.

Alpha hydroxy peel treatments can also help these pigmented areas. Because this type of pigmentation also is primarily due to genetic factors, this treatment can be an ongoing battle and many times does not substantially improve, but the pigmented areas can be covered with good camouflage makeup.

Circles and darkness caused by blood cell "diffusion" can be treated with a complex of ingredients using a combination of peptides and ingredients known as hydroxysuccinimide and chrysin. Hydroxysuccinimide binds the iron in the hemoglobin to prevent degradation and pigment formation, while chrysin, a flavone derived from passionflower, promotes production of natural enzymes that will break down the pigments. Peptides palmitoyl oligopeptide and palmitoyl tetrapeptide work by helping to tighten the tissue to reduce the chances of capillary leakage.

Getting plenty of sleep and reducing stress certainly seems to have a positive effect. Rest and exercise also have a rejuvenating effect on the skin, probably due to improved circulation and stress reduction.

**Q** Now that I am in my late 20s, my skin doesn't seem to be one color any more. It seems like it's frecklier than it was just a few years ago. Is there something I can do about this?

**A** This sounds like classic sun damage symptoms that would occur in the mid- to late 20s. The first visible sign of cumulative sun damage is often uneven pigment.

The first thing to do is start wearing a daily broad-spectrum sunscreen with an SPF of at least 15. Look for a sunscreen-moisturizer tailored for your specific skin type and that is comfortable on your skin. This can be used as a morning moisturizer or as a pre-makeup moisturizer. Make sure to use it *every day*! This step alone will make a difference in the appearance of your skin.

Additionally, the use of an alpha hydroxy serum once or twice a day will help remove dead surface cells that are already stained with pigment, helping to even out your skin tone. Lastly, and in addition to sunscreen and alpha hydroxy serum, use of a serum containing the antioxidant magnesium ascorbyl phosphate, a vitamin C derivative, can help to further suppress the splotchy pigment.

This treatment regime should be ongoing. Stopping use of the product will result in return of the uneven skin tone.

Salon alpha hydroxy peeling treatments will boost the effect of these products and help to speed the evening of the skin tone.

**Q** **I get red easily—my skin seems to react to things more than most people's skin. Are there things I should do or not do?**

**A** You definitely should consult a dermatologist and a licensed esthetician/skin therapist. There is a good chance you might have rosacea (see Chapter 4 on sensitive skin). Your dermatologist can diagnose this and may give you prescription topical treatment if your symptoms are severe.

In general, sensitive skin (including rosacea) should avoid exposure to any sort of heat, sun, and extreme temperature changes in general. Try to keep the skin as cool as possible, without being uncomfortable. Take warm instead of hot showers, allow hot cars to air out in the summer before getting in the car, and stay out of the sauna at the gym. Exercise does increase blood flow and body temperature and can cause flushing or flares in some people. It is best to exercise inside, in the pool, or outside in the cooler hours of the day with less sun exposure.

Regarding skin care, stay away from anything fragranced; anything with drying alcohols, rough exfoliators (including microdermabrasion), and stripping cleansers; or anything stimulating, including essential oils. Look for soothing, fragrance-free, irritancy-tested products. Lotions and fluids are usually better than creams for this skin. Be careful with exfoliators such as alpha hydroxy acids, which can be used on sensitive skin if they are formulated and used properly. Consult an experienced licensed skin therapist who is well trained in sensitive skin to help you choose the right products to use at home.

Food-wise, there are differences among redness-prone individuals. Not all redness-inducing foods affect everyone. That being said, the culprits may include alcohol (especially red wine), hot beverages, caffeine, citrus fruits and juices, and spicy foods. If you notice consistent reddening after eating or drinking a particular food or beverage, stay away from that food or beverage.

**Q** **Are there skin care products I should use that might help with the redness?**

**A** Besides avoiding the product types listed above, look for very gentle low-foaming cleansers, alcohol-free toners, and products that have been tested for sensitive skin. All products for your skin should be fragrance-free.

Products that include green tea, grapeseed, elizabethae (sea whip), licorice, or matricaria extracts may be helpful in soothing and reducing the redness. Some of the same ingredients used to treat dark circles, such as hesperidin methyl chalcone and dipeptide-2, may also be helpful in controlling redness. Products that help to supplement or reinforce the barrier function of the skin may be helpful as well. Barrier function problems are prevalent in skin with rosacea.

Generally speaking, the fewer products you use, the better off your skin will be. Three or four products should

be plenty to take care of your skin, without chancing flushing and redness.

**Q** **I have obvious capillaries on the sides of my nostrils. What causes these and how can I treat them?**

**A** These are distended capillaries known as telangiectasias. They are not actually broken but are enlarged to the point that they are easily seen. They tend to look worse when the skin is inflamed or hot. They also may be more prominent when the person drinks alcoholic beverages or has high blood pressure.

Using products designed for redness-prone skin may help their appearance to some degree. However, to make them completely disappear, they will need treatment by a medical professional with laser or other device to cut off the blood flow to these capillaries. For more information on this procedure, see Chapter 10.

**Q** **I have big, dark, red splotches on the sides of my neck. They almost look like a horseshoe pattern. What are these splotches?**

**A** It sounds like you have a symptom called **poikiloderma of Cevattes,** a symptom of severe cumulative sun dam-age. These areas of the neck have been chronically ex-posed, unprotected, to the sun. The pattern is caused by the way the sun has hit the contours of the neck. The area in the middle of the neck is lighter because it has been shaded from the sun by the natural structure of the face.

Over time, capillaries in this area have distended and heavy pigmentation has developed. These areas are a mix of redness and hyperpigmentation. There are often many obvious red capillaries throughout the splotchy areas. There may also be wrinkling and rough textures in the areas.

**Q.** Can anything be done to help the appearance of poikiloderma?

**A** You need the help of a skin care professional to design a program for your skin. A mix of alpha hydroxy acid, sunscreen, lipids, antioxidants, anti-redness ingredients, along with routine salon treatments, using a mix of light peels and LED light treatments, can help this.

   You need to understand that this much damage will not look better overnight. You must diligently perform your skin care program and follow the advice of a good skin care professional. It may take months of treatment to improve this problem.

**Q.** I had too much sun in my 20s and 30s and am now suffering the results. Can you recommend a regimen for my skin?

**A** You need to see a qualified skin care professional to develop a program that is specific to your individual skin condition. Having said that, here are the basic types of products you should be using:

**Morning**
- A foaming cleanser suited to your skin type that can easily be used in the shower. Keep water temperature to warm. Hot water or very cold water is not good for the skin.
- A toner, again chosen for your skin type. Toners that are in spray bottles are easiest to use.
- A soothing antioxidant or peptide serum to help with firmness and inflammation. This should be a lightweight fluid easily applied prior to your sunscreen/moisturizer.
- A combination sunscreen/moisturizer with an SPF of 15 or higher. This should be broad-spectrum with UVA and UVB screening ingredients, and again suited for your skin type. It is important that this product is the right weight for your skin and has the proper emollient level.

You should really like the feel of this product so you will use it consistently.

- An eye cream containing peptides, lipids, antioxidants, or other age-management ingredients. Again, this product should be chosen for you by a qualified esthetician or skin therapist. There are many eye products now available that help with puffiness, wrinkling, sagging, and darkness.

**Evening**

- Remove your makeup with a cleansing milk selected for your skin type.
- Repeat the toner you used in the morning.
- Reapply the peptide serum as you did in the morning.
- An alpha hydroxy acid product should be used. Specifically selected for your skin type, this product may be used twice a day for some heavier or more damaged skin types.
- A night hydrating and conditioning cream for your specific skin. This product is meant to increase the moisture level of your skin but may contain other conditioning ingredients such as firming or wrinkle-relaxing peptides, antiredness ingredients if needed, and antioxidants or lipids to improve barrier function.
- Eye cream should be repeated as in the morning routine.

**Q** How often should I clean my skin?

**A** Generally speaking, the skin should be cleansed twice a day—in the morning with a foaming or rinseable cleanser, and before bedtime with a cleansing milk to remove makeup.

This may vary if you do not wear makeup or have very dry or very oily skin. If you do not wear makeup, you may be able to use just a rinse-off cleanser twice a day. Very dry skin may need to avoid any foaming cleanser and stick to using nonfoaming cleansing milks at all times to avoid damaging the barrier function.

Very oily skin may need an additional cleansing in the afternoon to control oiliness. People with oily skin may also require stronger cleansers to control oiliness.

Never cleanse the skin more than three times a day, even if you have extremely oily skin. Too much cleansing can cause dryness, inflammation, and redness; worsen some forms of acne; and accentuate wrinkles and symptoms of aging.

**Q** What is the best way to remove facial hair?

**A** There are three main types of hair removal procedures used by professionals:

Waxing is a temporary but fast and inexpensive way to remove unwanted facial hair. Depilatory wax is applied with a spatula and removed quickly, removing the hair from the bottom of the follicle. There are several different types of wax-type products. Your skin therapist will choose the right one for your skin type and the area being waxed. After waxing, your skin may be red for up to a day, but usually for only an hour or two. Some people do not experience any redness. The skin therapist should apply a soothing fluid after waxing that should help to make the area feel better and reduce redness faster.

**Electrolysis** is a technique that treats individual hairs with electrical current, heat, or both to kill the growth cells of the hair in the base of the follicle. A fine needle called a filament is inserted into the follicle and electricity is released down the filament. Galvanic current causes the formation of a "destructive" chemical in the follicle (electrolysis), and short wave, a different type of current, creates heat in a process called **thermolysis.** There is a technique called the **blend** that uses a blend of both techniques. Each individual hair must be treated, often more than once, to destroy all the growth cells in each follicle.

Electrolysis is a good choice for thick, stiff chin hairs and lip areas, but it can be used anywhere on the body.

**Laser hair removal** uses laser and light to damage the growth cells. This technique is especially effective for larger areas such as backs or legs, but it can be expensive and must be repeated many times. In most states, this technique must be performed or supervised by licensed medical professionals.

**Q** **What is the best way to find a good esthetician or skin therapist?**

**A** This is a good question. In most states, estheticians, also sometimes called facial specialists, skin care specialists, or skin therapists, are regulated by the State Board of Cosmetology. Many states have websites so consumers can check to make sure their specialist is licensed.

The education level of estheticians and the amount of education required for licensure by individual states can vary greatly. Most estheticians who have additional certifications from skin care associations or additional degrees are generally better choices.

There are also estheticians that concentrate more on pampering and relaxation, and others who specialize in corrective skin care. These corrective estheticians focus more on skin problems and programs to achieve real change in the skin's appearance.

Experience certainly counts, and skin care salons or clinics that have been in business for many years are generally good choices. Check with your local Better Business Bureau. They will have success and complaint records of registered skin care facilities.

Probably the best way to find a good esthetician is by word of mouth or reputation. Ask neighbors, friends, or your physician or dermatologist.

It is certainly acceptable to visit a salon or clinic for a tour. Look for cleanliness, accreditations, and professionalism in the staff. It is also a good idea to schedule a consultation before starting a treatment program. You may have to pay for a consultation, but you can get the opinion of the therapist and decide for yourself if he or she is the right choice.

**Q** **I have never had a professional facial treatment before. What are the basics of a professional facial?**

**A** Your first treatment should begin with you filling out a health history form. This is primarily to check for allergies and contraindications—skin care procedures that should be avoided based on your health condition or prescription drugs. It will help your skin therapist design a better program for your skin.

All treatments begin with skin cleansing. Your makeup will be removed and your facial skin thoroughly cleansed using cleansing lotion with sponges or cotton pads. After the skin is completely clean, the therapist will examine your skin carefully with a lighted magnifying loop. The therapist may ask you questions about your skin's behavior, and may ask more detailed questions about previous skin treatment. This procedure is called skin analysis, and it is during the analysis that your skin type and skin conditions are determined. The therapist will use this information to design your facial treatment plan, as well as choose your home care product regimen.

After the analysis, the therapist will begin a series of procedures based on your condition. These may include the following:

- Steam treatment is used to hydrate the skin surface, loosen dead cells, and soften skin for further cleansing. Steam may be warm or cold depending on your sensitivity level.
- Exfoliation helps to remove surface dead cells and further cleanse the skin. A rotating brush may be used to

gently exfoliate the skin. This step may be omitted in sensitive skin types. Some therapists will use a chemical exfoliation procedure such as an enzyme peel or a mechanical product such as a mild granular scrub or sloughing product instead of brushing.

- For oily or clogged skin, a procedure called desincrustation may be performed. This procedure uses a specialized product to soften pore impactions. Sometimes a mild galvanic current may be used to help penetrate this product.

- The softened impactions are then removed using a technique called extraction. Extraction is a manual procedure in which the therapist manipulates the skin with cotton-covered fingers, cotton swabs, and sometimes an instrument called a comedo extractor. Extraction expels the content of individual follicles, removing clogged pores. If you have many clogged pores, not all will be removed in the first visit. Your therapist will recommend the correct home care products to improve this condition. After extraction, a serum will be applied to help prevent inflammation.

- Massage is the part of the treatment that most people think of when they think of a facial. Massage is relaxing but is also good for the skin in terms of stimulating circulation, and also beneficial in helping to penetrate conditioning products. Massage may be avoided in clients with very oily skin or acne problems.

- Electrical treatment may be used to stimulate or help penetrate products. The two most popular electrical treatments are known as high frequency and ionization. High frequency uses a "buzzing" glass electrode to stimulate the skin, and it helps to kill surface bacteria after extraction. Another electrical treatment called ionization often uses metal rollers for product penetration.

- A mask or masks are chosen to complete the facial treatment. These will be determined by the therapist, based on your skin type, condition, and your skin response during the previous procedures. Masks are used to tone, hydrate, cleanse, or soothe the skin.

- After relaxing with the mask treatment for 10–20 minutes, the mask is removed, and a moisturizer and sunscreen are applied.
- Many therapists ask their clients to avoid makeup for an hour or two after a facial treatment. This helps avoid inflammation, and many therapists believe that the treatment will show better results if makeup is not worn immediately after the treatment.
- Other procedures such as hand treatments, brow arching, or facial waxing may be performed in conjunction with the facial, depending on the salon and your needs.
- Finally, the skin therapist will consult with you and will explain what program he or she believes will benefit your skin. Home care product procedures as well as professional treatment recommendations will be made.

**Q** **How often should I have a professional facial treatment?**

**A** This depends on your skin condition and what you are trying to achieve. Keep in mind that all skin care programs must be performed consistently to be truly effective. This includes both home care as well as professional treatment.

If you have problem skin, acne, or aging issues, you may be advised to have a series of treatments, usually one per week or one every two weeks. The type of treatments advised depend on your skin problems. For example, microcurrent treatments designed to tighten the appearance of the skin must be done in a series to be effective. Twice-a-week treatments with microcurrent are typical when beginning treatment. Once the desired results are achieved, you must keep up the treatments in monthly or twice-monthly frequency to keep the results. The same is true for alpha hydroxy peels or LED treatments. All of these treatments must be performed in series to be effective.

Once the desired results have been achieved, once-a-month professional treatment is advisable for many clients. Again, this will vary with your skin type.

Don't forget that the most important part of any skin care program is performing the right home care on a consistent daily basis. Only with consistent home care can the best results be achieved.

# CHAPTER 10

# Problems That Need a Doctor

**AUTHOR'S NOTE**

This chapter is not meant to diagnose or to prescribe medical treatment for any skin or medical condition. It is simply meant to provide basic education and information about common skin problems that require diagnosis by a qualified physician.

If you have any skin condition that does not respond to home care, please seek the advice of a qualified physician.

**Q** My acne never seems to completely clear. I constantly have pimples on my chin and jaw line. What do you suggest?

**A** Chronic acne in the chin and jaw line area in women may indicate hormone imbalances that require medical treatment. This is particularly true when the acne does not respond to topical treatment. It is a fairly common problem among younger women. Medical treatment involves hormone-based prescription medication, which may help clear this chronic acne problem. There are types of birth control pills also available that help to control these imbalances that aggravate acne-prone skin.

If you have tried the skin care recommendations made in the problem skin chapter and still are not seeing substantial improvement in the chin and jaw line area, make an appointment with a dermatologist or your family doctor for consultation.

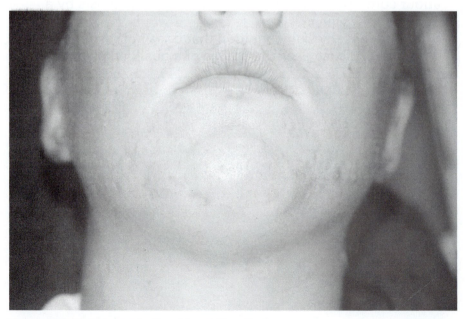

Hormonal-related acne in the chin and jaw line.

**Q** I have had a lot of problems with hormones, which has affected not only my acne-prone skin but also caused pigment problems (melasma). Is there a type of doctor who specializes in just hormone-related problems?

**A** Yes. A physician who specializes in hormone problems is an **endocrinologist.** Endocrinologists can provide specialized help for people who have constant hormone fluctuations. They are a good choice for help, especially when other routes have already been taken.

**Q** I have oily skin and have several little places that look like blackheads, but there is nothing in them. Some are shaped like little donuts. What are these?

**A** These are most likely **sebaceous hyperplasias,** which are overgrown sebaceous glands that are pressing upwards on the tissue around the follicle, creating a ridge around the follicle opening. They occur only on the face, usually in oilier areas, and are often mistaken for open comedones (blackheads). They can occur in different sizes and tend to grow if not treated. Although they are a nuisance and not attractive, they are not indicative of any serious skin condition.

No one knows the cause of sebaceous hyperplasias, but they are thought to be possibly associated with sun damage. They are much more likely to occur in persons with oily skin who are over 30 years of age.

**Q** Can sebaceous hyperplasias be treated?

**A** There is no home care treatment to correct hyperplasias. Likewise, they are generally not affected by topical facial treatments.

Dermatologists treat sebaceous hyperplasias with several different methods:

- For small hyperplasias, they may be treated with cryosurgery (liquid nitrogen), which freezes the surface tissue, which eventually falls off the skin.

- Because the sebaceous glands are located deep in the dermis, sometimes dermatologists will insert a small filament needle into the follicle and attach the needle to a machine called a hyfrecator, better known as an electric needle. The current travels down the needle and kills some of the cells in the sebaceous gland. This will eventually causes a flattening effect on the skin surface.
- Lasers may also be used to treat these lesions.
- Larger lesions may need to be removed surgically.

People who get sebaceous hyperplasias tend to get more than one. The sebaceous glands are never completely destroyed and often will start to overgrow again, even after they have been treated. So, even though the lesions can be treated to look better, they may reoccur.

It is best to treat sebaceous hyperplasias when they are still small. Removing larger hyperplasias surgically is much more likely to leave visible scars than treating small hyperplasias with cryosurgery, hyfrecation, or laser.

**Q** I get these little red pimples around my chin and mouth. It looks like acne, and the bumps appear in little groups. They do not respond to benzoyl peroxide or any topical treatment. What might these bumps be?

**A** Clusters of papules around the mouth area may be indicative of a condition known as **perioral dermatitis,** which literally means skin inflammation around the mouth. Although it most often occurs in the chin area, it can also occur above the lips, in the nasalabial folds, and on the cheeks.

A key sign of this condition is the cluster pattern of the papules, occurring in little "groups."

Perioral dermatitis occurs almost exclusively in women in their early 20s through their mid- to late 40s. The cause of perioral dermatitis is unknown, but it has been theorized to be hormonal in nature and also has been

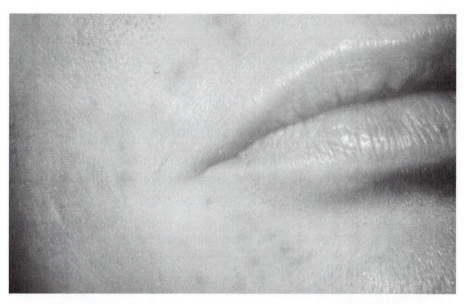

Perioral dermatitis appears in clusters of papules around the mouth area *(courtesy Mark Lees Skin Care, Inc.)*.

associated with fluoride toothpaste and overuse of moisturizers (although neither of these has been proven).

Perioral dermatitis must be treated with oral antibiotics such as tetracycline for several weeks. Topical treatment, including topical antibiotics, or discontinuation of home care is ineffective. Discontinuation of any heavy moisturization and avoidance of fragranced or stimulating skin care products is often advised, in tandem with the oral antibiotic treatment.

**Q** **Every change of season, I get red, flaky skin around my hairline, the sides and corners of my nose, and sometimes in my eyebrows. Can you tell me what this might be?**

**A** There are many medical conditions that might fit this description, but because of the location of the flaking, it is most likely **seborrheic dermatitis.** Seborrheic dermatitis is a common condition that is an inflammation of the sebaceous glands that results in inflamed, red, and flaky skin.

It typically occurs in oilier areas of the face, such as the nose and T-zone. Flaking and redness in the eyebrows is a frequent sign of seborrheic dermatitis. The ears and scalp are also affected. It is often a chronic condition and may

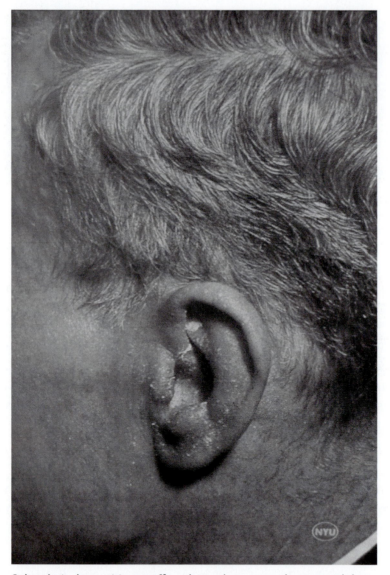

Seborrheic dermatitis can affect the scalp, ears, eyebrows, and the T-zone of the face *(Reprinted with permission from the American Academy of Dermatology. All rights reserved.)*.

return frequently after being treated. It is not known why change of season or, more specifically, change of weather seems to flare seborrheic dermatitis, but it is theorized to be related to changes in humidity.

People make the mistake of thinking that the condition is dry skin and treat it with heavy moisturizers, which can actually make the condition more inflamed.

Seborrheic dermatitis, especially if chronic, is best managed by a dermatologist. The exact cause of seborrheic dermatitis is unknown but is thought to be related to yeast on the skin. It is treated with anti-yeast pharmaceutical topical creams containing an active ingredient called ketaconazole. Topical hydrocortisone is also used to control the inflammation.

**Q** **Are there skin care modifications that should take place for seborrheic dermatitis?**

**A** Lightweight, non-comedogenic, and nonfragranced moisturizers may be helpful without aggravating the inflammation. Avoid alcohol-based skin care products, all stimulating products, and anything fragranced. While inflamed, avoid exfoliants and alpha hydroxy products and peels.

Cleanse the skin with a mild wash or cleansing milk. Harsh cleansers may make the inflammation worse. Toners containing drying alcohols may also inflame the condition.

When the skin has cleared, make sure to stick to the same basic rules, although the use of mild exfoliation and alpha hydroxy products may be resumed. Rich creams should always be avoided in seborrheic dermatitis patients.

Seborrheic dermatitis can be affected or worsened by some skin care but will not clear solely with skin care modifications. As stated above, seborrheic dermatitis must be treated with anti-yeast cream and topical hydrocortisone. A dermatologist should see chronic seborrheic dermatitis or conditions that do not clear with over-the-counter treatment. Rarely, seborrheic dermatitis can be indicative of other internal diseases.

**Q** **I have a little red bump on my nose that keeps coming back. Sometimes it flakes. Once in a while it will bleed when I wash my face. What should I do about this bump?**

**A** This type of lesion always needs to be checked by a dermatologist. Any unexplained bleeding anywhere on or in the body should be promptly seen by a physician.

There are types of skin precancers and cancers that can seem to come and go, but they never really go away. Flaking may be one symptom of a skin cancer. A patient will treat the lesion with moisturizer; the flaking will stop; the patient will think the lesion went away; and then, of course, it comes back. Again, any reoccurring lesion anywhere on the body should be promptly checked by a doctor.

Neglecting a skin cancer can lead to the need for much more invasive treatment. The faster a cancer is diagnosed, the simpler the treatment in general, and this lessens the risk of scarring. If you have any unexplained lesion, please see a dermatologist and have it checked.

**Q** **What does skin cancer look like?**

**A** There are various types of skin cancer, but the most common are the following:

- **Basal cell carcinomas**—the most common type of skin cancer—often appear as small pearl-like bumps, and sometimes has tiny visible capillaries running through it. Occasionally it will appear as a reoccurring

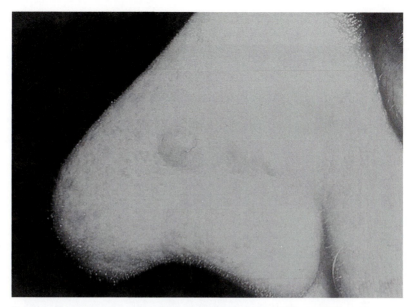

Basal cell carcinoma sometimes looks like a pearl-like nodule
(courtesy Rube J. Pardo, M.D., Ph.D.).

pimple (see above). In their early stages, basal cell carcinomas sometimes look like white, flat scars on the skin.

- **Squamous cell carcinomas** tend to look like crusty bumps and can vary in size. They are usually raised. Early squamous cell carcinomas can look like a crusty patch of skin. They are more aggressive than basal cell carcinomas and can rarely metastasize. Squamous cell carcinomas are more likely to occur in men than women, occurring on the face, lips, ears, and on any sun-exposed skin surface.
- **Melanoma**—the most deadly form of skin cancer—is characterized by unusual-looking moles or lesions that look like moles. There are five characteristics of melanomas to identify suspicious lesions that need dermatological help. They are known as the **ABCDEs of melanoma.**

  - **A** stands for asymmetry. The two sides of the lesion are not alike.

- **B** stands for border. The border or edges of the lesion are uneven or jagged.
- **C** stands for color. Melanomas are often more than one color, and can be a mix of black, brown, purplish, and sometimes deep red.

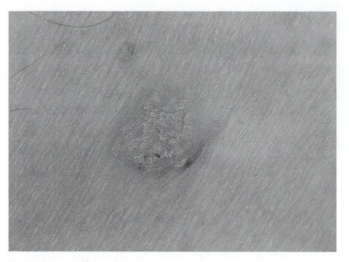

Squamous cell carcinoma *(courtesy Michael J. Bond, M.D.).*

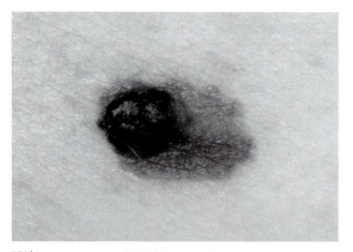

Melanoma *(courtesy of The Skin Cancer Foundation, www.skincancer.org).*

- **D** stands for diameter, about that of a pencil eraser or larger.
- **E** stands for evolving. The lesion can change, and you may notice differences in the lesion over even a short time.

The earlier any skin cancer is detected and diagnosed, the better the odds of cure and recovery. If you have a suspicious lesion that looks odd, even if it does not match the descriptions of cancer appearance exactly, have it checked by a dermatologist. It is always better to get something checked than to ignore a possible problem condition, especially when it comes to skin cancer!

Both basal and squamous cell carcinomas are treatable, especially when treated and diagnosed early. They are treated by surgical removal, by scraping with a scoop-like surgical tool called a **curette,** followed by **electrodessication** or burning the scooped-out area of the lesion with an electric needle called a hyfrecator.

Melanoma, depending on the stage of the cancer, may be treated surgically, with radiation or with chemotherapy, or with a combination of these modalities.

**Q** I am 60 years old and I have some areas on my face and hands that are red and so dry the skin feels prickly, almost like it has little sharp bumps. What are these?

**A** These could also be a precancerous area known as **actinic keratosis.** Red, dry, flaky areas in skin that has been repeatedly sun exposed are likely to be this sun damage symptom. Actinic keratosis is prevalent in lighter skins, especially of Celtic or western European descent. They frequently occur on the face, especially the forehead, upper cheeks, and temples, and on the hands and arms.

Persons who have actinic keratosis should be checked for skin cancer thoroughly and often by a qualified

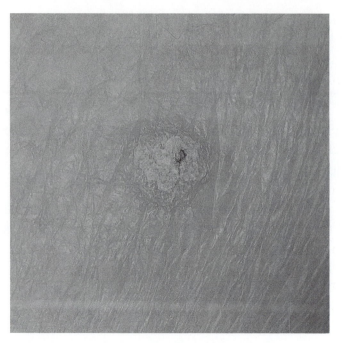

Actinic keratosis feels rough and prickly and does not clear like dry skin *(courtesy Michael J. Bond, M.D.).*

dermatologist. Actinic keratosis is often treated with cryo-surgery (freezing the lesion).

Sometimes, in cases where there are many lesions or large areas of lesions, a drug therapy called Efudex is used. This chemical peel-like drug is applied at home. This will help to clear multiple actinic keratoses, but it does cause a lot of irritation during the therapy. Again, this type of therapy should be administered under the supervision of a dermatologist who can also help with the irritation symptoms.

**Q** I have flat, yellowish bumps around my eyes. What might they be?

**A** This should be checked by a dermatologist for proper diagnosis, but these lesions sound like small skin pockets

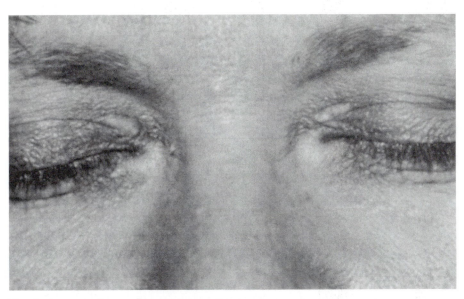

Xanthelasmas often occur on the eyelids *(courtesy Timothy G. Berger, M.D.)*.

of cholesterol called **xanthelasmas.** Xanthelasmas occur predominantly in older skin, often sun damaged. They may or may not be related to high blood cholesterol levels.

Xanthelasmas are frequently seen in the upper and lower lid areas and are often egg-shaped and yellowish-white in color. Xanthelasmas are most effectively treated with laser.

**Q** **I am 65 years old and have a large, flat, crusty-looking spot on my cheekbone. Can you tell me what you think this might be?**

**A** Again, this should be seen by a dermatologist for official diagnosis, but it could likely be a sun-damage lesion known as a **seborrheic keratosis.** This is basically a pileup of cells that appear in a patch-like, slightly raised lesion. They often look like gray or flesh-colored scabs, almost as if they are "stuck" on the skin surface. They are frequently found on sun-exposed body areas such as faces and hands, but they can appear anywhere on the body in a sun-damaged skin. They are mostly an esthetic nuisance but are indicative of cumulative sun damage.

Dermatologists can remove seborrheic keratoses (plural) by scraping them off with a specialized surgical tool.

**Q** **What causes enlarged capillaries?**

**A** Enlarged or distended capillaries, medically known as telangiectasias, are obvious small red blood vessels. Primarily seen on the face, the vessels can also occur on the chest and other areas. Telangiectasias are frequently seen on the nose and cheeks.

The tendency to develop telangiectasias is hereditary, but sun exposure, alcohol and tobacco use, rosacea, and high blood pressure can play roles in their development.

**Q** **What medical treatment options are available for enlarged capillaries?**

**A** Telangiectasias are primarily an esthetic nuisance but can be signs of other problems such as rosacea.

Traditionally, they are treated by hyfrecation (with an electric needle) that cuts off the blood flow to the vessel.

Nowadays, telangiectasias are more effectively treated with specialized vascular lasers, which quickly cause their disappearance. Even larger areas can be treated. There is little risk of scarring from treatment and, in most cases, it does not require any downtime.

Because the formation of telangiectasias is hereditary, the lesions will often reoccur and must be retreated.

**Q** **If a person has had a lot of sun over his or her lifetime, how often should he or she have a dermatologist's checkup?**

**A** Annual skin checkups are advised for most adults. For persons who have had a lot of cumulative sun exposure or have had skin cancers treated, checkups may be advised more often. Ask your dermatologist how often he or she advises for you.

Early detection of any kind of cancer, including skin cancers, increases chances of recovery and lessens chances of scarring.

A good skin cancer check will entail the medical inspection of every part of the body, including the genitalia, and even the soles of the feet, scalp, and toenails.

It is also advised that every person also perform a thorough self-exam of the skin, using mirrors or having a partner check you, on a regular basis. This practice should be in addition to regular dermatologist's checkups.

**Q** **Are there effective treatments now available for birthmarks?**

**A** This is an area of medicine that has made huge strides in progress with the advent of laser surgery. Lasers can be used to remove several types of birthmarks including pigmented lesions and vascular birthmarks such as port-wine stains.

Laser treatment will vary with the lesion and should be administered by a board-certified dermatologist or plastic surgeon.

**Q** **I have scars from acne. What can be done about these?**

**A** There are two types of scarring: hypotrophic and hypertrophic. Hypotrophic scarring results in depressions or pockmarks in the skin. The skin surface is depressed in the area of scarring. This is typical of long-term acne scarring. Raised scars are hypertrophic scars. Sometimes these are also present in acne scarring.

If scar tissue is treated early when it is first forming, steroid injections can sometimes be used. These injections help to stop the formation of the scar as well as soften any scar tissue that has already formed.

Existing scars must be treated by removing dermal tissue, which is where the scar tissue is actually located. This can be accomplished by using an ablative laser, which works by vaporizing tissue. This is the type of laser that is often used by plastic surgeons and dermatologists to plane down wrinkling around the mouth and eyes. Another procedure, **dermabrasion,** is a surgical technique that uses a rotating wire brush to "sand down" skin tissue, removing layers of scar tissue. Dermabrasion used to be the standard for treating acne scarring, but laser is now generally the preferred technique because the amount of tissue and specific areas of tissue removed is more specific.

**Q** Can microdermabrasion help with acne scarring?

**A** Microdermabrasion can make the skin surface look smoother, but microdermabrasion is not deep enough to affect scar tissue, which is located in the dermis. To affect the dermis, a laser or surgical dermabrasion device, as discussed above, must be used. This should only be performed by a board certified dermatologist or plastic surgeon.

**Q** What are the differences between peels I get from my esthetician and peels I might get from a plastic surgeon?

**A** There are three types or levels of chemical peeling treatments:

- Superficial peels, also sometimes called micro-peels, "lunchtime peels," or exfoliating treatments, affect or remove dead cells only from the epidermis, the outer general layer of the skin. These include alpha hydroxy and glycolic acid peels, beta hydroxy (salicylic acid) peels, enzyme peels, Jessner's peels, and Unna peels. These treatments vary in strength and aggression in peeling, but they all only affect the epidermis. Superficial peels are the only types of peels that should be performed by experienced estheticians.

- Medium depth peels affect and remove the entire epidermis and some of the dermal tissue. The typical chemical used for this procedure is **trichloroacetic acid (TCA).** TCA is used at different concentrations, depending on the depth of peel desired. Lower-strength TCA peels are sometimes administered by estheticians, but higher-concentrated TCA peels should only be done by a board certified dermatologist or plastic surgeon.

- Deep or **surgical peels** use a chemical called phenol, a strong peeling agent. This peel is used for very wrinkled, extremely sun-damaged skin to smooth out multiple wrinkles. Phenol peeling has its risks, including the possibility of scarring, hypopigmentation (white splotching), and hyperpigmentation. The procedure is also quite painful and takes weeks to properly recover. Phenol is a chemical that can be absorbed and affect the heart, and it must be carefully administered by an experienced, board certified dermatologist or plastic surgeon. It is often applied in small areas because of the absorption risk.

# GLOSSARY

## A

**ablative (ah-blay-tiv)**  devices or techniques such as lasers that are used to remove surface skin tissue

**absorbing screen ingredients**  absorb and neutralize UV rays; also sometimes wrongly referred to as chemical screens (which is inaccurate, because all sunscreens are chemicals)

**acetyl hexapeptide-3 (ah-seat-al hex-ah-pep-tide)**  commercially known as Argireline—works by inhibiting certain binding proteins that create the tension that causes wrinkling

**Accutane**  an oral prescription retinoid drug used to treat cystic acne

**acne excoriée (ex-core-ee-ay)**  the medical term for acne that has been excoriated, which means scratched or scraped

**acnegenic**  describes a reaction or product that causes inflammation within the follicle resulting in follicular swelling and causing overnight pimples or acne flares

**actinic keratosis**  a precancerous area characterized by red, dry, flaky areas that may feel prickly to the touch in skin that has been repeatedly sun-exposed; they frequently occur on the face, especially the forehead, upper cheeks, and temples, and on the hands and arms

**adrenaline**  a hormone produced by the adrenal gland to cope with stress or emergencies

**allergy**  the body's immune system rejecting a particular substance

**allergens**  substances that trigger allergic reactions

**alipidic**  dry skin caused by skin that is not producing enough sebum

**alpha hydroxy acids (AHAs)**  family of naturally occurring mild acids used as exfoliants and hydrators; AHAs include glycolic, lactic, tartaric, malic, and mandelic acids

**ambient sun exposure**   unintentional exposure to the sun during typical daylight activities

**anaerobic**   describes bacteria, including *P. acnes* bacteria, that only survive in the absence of oxygen

**androgens**   male hormones

**antioxidants**   natural substances that prevent oxidation or neutralize free radicals in the skin or body, which cause inflammation and interfering with normal cellular functioning

**arbutin**   performance agent used in "skin brightening" products, but are not, at this time, FDA-approved for over-the-counter use as a skin lightening agent

**ascorbyl palmitate**   ester form of vitamin C

# B

**barrier function**   refers to the complex of lipids (fatty materials) that are present between the cells in the corneum, which guards moisture (transepidermal water loss—TEWL) and protects against dehydration, and also provides a lipid barrier to prevent irritants from entering the skin

**basal cells**   lowest level of cells in the epidermis where new epidermal skin cells are produced

**basal cell carcinomas**   the most common type of skin cancer, often appears as small pearl-like bumps and sometimes has tiny visible capillaries running through it

**basal layer**   the lowest layer of the epidermis

**bearberry extract**   performance agent used in "skin brightening" products, but are not, at this time, FDA-approved for over-the-counter use as a skin lightening agent

**beta hydroxy acids (BHAs)**   naturally occurring mild acids used for exfoliation, soothing, and as an antibacterial; includes the widely used salicylic acid

**biologically inert**   an ingredient that does not cross-react with chemicals in the body

**blepharoplasty (blef-ah-ro-plastee)**   a plastic surgery eyelift

**broad-spectrum antioxidant**   a product that contains numerous antioxidants to squelch a variety of oxidative reactions

**broad-spectrum sunscreen**   sunscreen that filters both UVA and UVB rays

# C

**carotenoids**   yellow pigments from certain foods such as carrots

**chemical exfoliation**   the use of a product that dissolves or loosens dead cell buildup

**closed comedones**   sebum- and dead cell–impacted follicles with tiny follicle openings

**collagen**   an abundant protein present in the reticular dermis that gives firmness to the skin

**collagenase**   an enzyme the skin makes that breaks up excess collagen

**combination skin**   facial skin with a mix of oily and dry areas

**comedogenic**   describes agents or products that cause comedones to develop

**comedogenicity**   the tendency of a topical agent or product to cause clogged pores and comedones to develop

**comedone extractors**   instruments that assist in the extraction of comedones from the skin

**corneocytes**   keratinocytes in the stratum corneum layer

**couperose**   European term describing areas with distended capillaries

**curette**   a scoop-like surgical tool frequently used to surgically remove skin cancers

**cystic acne**   a severe form of acne in which the skin forms deep pockets of infection

# D

**deep peels**   also sometimes called surgical peels, performed only by dermatologists and plastic surgeons, removes the entire epidermis and also removes dermal tissue

**dehydrated skin**   skin lacking water or moisture, resulting in flaking, tightness, itching, and sometimes stinging and burning

**dermabrasion**   a surgical technique that uses a rotating wire brush to "sand down" skin tissue, removing layers of scar tissue

**dendrites**   branch-like extensions on the ends of certain cells

**dendritic**   describes cells that have tentacle-like branches

**depigmentation**   the process of using drugs to destroy pigment in the skin; used to even out skin color in cases of vitiligo

**dermatoheliosis**   the medical term for skin damage from sun exposure

**dermis**   the live layer of skin under the epidermis

**desincrustation** a technique or product that helps to liquefy or loosen solidified sebum impacted in follicles or comedones

**detergents** surfactants used as cleansing agents in foaming cleansers

**dihydroxyacetone (die-hydroxy-as-ah-tone)** an ingredient used in sunless tanning and spray tans, which causes keratin proteins in epidermal cells to darken

**dipeptide-2** peptide ingredient used for eye puffiness

**dipotassium glycyrrhizinate (die-potassium gly-sir-riz-inate)** derived from licorice; a strong antioxidant used in products to curb irritancy

## E

**elastin** a protein within the reticular dermis that gives flexibility and elasticity to the skin

**elastosis** medical term for skin sagging

**electrodessication** purposeful medical destruction of tissue such as cancer by burning the lesion with an electric needle called a hyfrecator

**electrolysis** a technique that treats individual hairs with electrical current, heat, or both to kill the growth cells of the hair in the base of the follicle

**elizabethae (sea whip) extract** extracted from coral and is a potent skin calmer

**emollients** ingredients that lie across the skin, often oils or fatty materials, helping to retain moisture and prevent dehydration

**endocrinologist** a physician who specializes in hormone problems

**epidermal-dermal junction** the area where the two main layers of the skin connect

**epidermis** the outermost layer of the skin

**ergocalciferol** vitamin D, involved in the skin in cell renewal, and may have many more functions

**estrogen** female hormone

**expression lines** facial wrinkles caused by repeated facial expressions

**extraction** the removal of debris and impactions from the follicles

**extrinsic skin aging** skin aging caused by sun exposure and environmental factors

**eumelanin (you-melanin)** a brown-black melanin pigment

## F

**fibroblasts** specialized cells that produce collagen

**Fitzpatrick Skin Typing** a measurement scale called that classifies skin coloration into six different skin color categories, indicating natural resistance to sun exposure, tendency to burn, and tendency to sun-related aging damage

**flares** periods of time when skin with rosacea has obvious symptoms and inflammation

**flushing** sudden reddening of the facial skin from sudden increased blood flow

**follicle** a duct in the skin that contains a hair and is attached to the sebaceous glands that produce sebum

**free radicals** unstable atoms that rob electrons from cells in the skin and can cause DNA damage to the cells and the fibroblasts that produce collagen; also produce biochemical damage that can lead to eventual skin cancers and abnormal growths

## G

**galvanic current** a type of electrical current used in the process of desincrustation to treat clogged pores or acne; also can be used in a process called iontophoressis, which helps to penetrate treatment products into the skin

**glycosaminoglycans (gly-cos-ameeno-gly-cans)** water-binding biochemicals in the reticular dermis that hold tremendous amounts of water

**grapeseed extract** strong antioxidant ingredients used in both aging and calming skin care products

**green tea extract** powerful antioxidant complex used in both aging and calming skin care products

**ground substance** a filler-like substance within the reticular dermis that helps the dermis retain moisture

## H

**helix** describes a ropelike braid; used to describe the structure of collagen

**high frequency current** specialized electrical cosmetic skin treatment used to stimulate blood flow and reduce surface bacteria, swelling, and inflammation; also helps with penetration of treatment products

**humectants** also known as **hydrophilic agents** or **hydrators,** skin care ingredients that help to attract water and bind the moisture to the cells and between the epidermal cells

**hyaluronic acid** an ingredient well known in moisturizers that holds 1,000 times its own weight in water; a component within the ground substance

**hydrators** see **humectants**

**hydrophilic agents** see **humectants**

**hydroquinone** a topical drug ingredient that is the most commonly used melanin suppressant

**hyperpigmentation** dark, splotchy areas of the skin where melanocytes in the skin have overproduced melanin

**hypertrophic scars** raised scars

**hypopigmentation** lack of pigment in the skin resulting in light spots

**hypotrophic scars** depressed (sunken) scars, which often are called pockmarks

## I

**inflammation cascade** also known as the free radical cascade, a domino effect of biochemical reactions that cause inflammation and eventual skin damage for sun exposure

**intense pulsed light (IPL)** a form of light therapy used by physicians to treat distended capillaries, hyperpigmentation, and perform hair reduction

**intercellular lipid matrix or intercellular cement** lipids between the cells in the corneum

**intrinsic skin aging** refers to aging of the skin that occurs naturally

## K

**keloid** hypertrophic scar that does not resolve because the skin hereditarily does not make collagen in a normal way

**keratin** a protein that fills the cells in the epidermis; also present in nails and hair

**keratinization** the process in which epidermal cells fill with keratin protein and migrate toward the epidermal corneum

**keratinocytes** cells going through the process of keratinization

**keratolytic** protein-dissolving; describes exfoliating agents used to remove dead cell buildup from the skin

**kojic acid** performance agent used in "skin brightening" products but not, at this time, FDA-approved for over-the-counter use as a skin lightening agent

# L

**l-ascorbic acid** acid form of vitamin C

**lamellar bodies** grainy-looking cells within the granular layer that produce lipids for the barrier function

**Langerhans cells (lawn-gur-hawns)** immune function cells that "patrol" the epidermis to detect foreign invaders or pathogens

**laser hair removal** uses laser and light to damage the growth cells of the hair

**lichochalcone (like-o-cal-cone)** derived from licorice; a strong antioxidant used in products to curb irritancy

**light emitting diodes (LED)** intense flashing light rays used by estheticians to treat appearance signs of aging, redness, acne, and other conditions

**lipid peroxide** a type of free radical caused when lipids are attacked in the cell membrane by other free radicals

**liposomes** tiny encapsulation vessels that are often filled with performance skin care ingredients

# M

**magnesium ascorbyl phosphate** an ester form of topical vitamin C used as an antioxidant and brightening agent to help reduce the appearance of dark spots

**matricaria extract (matt-trick-care-ee-ah)** a type of chamomile extract frequently used in calming products

**mechanical exfoliation** removes surface cells by physically "bumping them off" the skin

**medium depth peels** performed using trichloroacetic acid, removes the entire epidermis and also removes some dermal tissue; only a dermatologist or plastic surgeon should perform this peel

**melanin** skin pigment that causes skin color and tanning

**melanin suppressant** a topical substance that interferes with the biochemical process that produces melanin in skin cells

**melanocytes** pigment-producing cells that are found in both the lower epidermis and the dermis

**melanoma**   the most deadly form of skin cancer; characterized by unusual-looking moles or lesions that look like moles

**melanosomes**   granules of pigment produced by melanocytes

**melasma**   hyperpigmentation associated with hormonal influence; also sometimes called pregnancy mask, a pattern of a mask affecting the forehead, cheeks, chin, and upper lip

**micro-current**   a gentle electrical current applied to the skin with probes, primarily used to improve the appearance of elastosis and aging, but can be used to help many different skin problems

**microcomedo**   the beginning of a comedo forming inside the base of follicle characterized by microscopic clumping of cell buildup

**mitotic division**   a biological process in which cells divide

# N

**nasolabial folds**   describes the area of the face from the corners of the mouth to the nose

# O

**objective symptoms**   visible and often measurable symptoms such as redness and flaking

**oil-dry or alipidic skin**   skin that is not producing enough protective sebum to prevent surface dehydration

**oily skin**   skin characterized by large, visible pores all across the skin, including the skin near the ears; the larger pores are due to the follicles being expanded to accommodate the large amount of sebum flowing through them

**open comedones**   a hardened mass of fatty materials in a follicle, mixed with dead cells from the hyperkeratosis; often called blackheads

**ostium**   follicle opening

# P

**palmitoyl oligopeptide (palm-ih-toyl ah-lih-go-pep-tide)**   peptide ingredients used to improve firmness

**palmitoyl pentapeptide-3**   commercially known as Matrixyl; helps to improve firmness of the skin

**palmitoyl tetrapeptide**   peptide ingredients used to improve firmness

**panthenol**   vitamin B5, used as a moisturizing ingredient in moisturizers

**papillary dermis**   the top layer within the dermis that connects the dermis to the epidermis

**papule**   a raised lesion characterized by redness; in acne, papules are "headless" red lesions (pimples) and tend to be sore

**peptides**   chains of amino acids theorized to send signals or somehow stimulate the skin to behave in a different way

**perioral dermatitis**   an acne-like condition characterized by clusters of papules around the mouth area and can also occur above the lips, in the nasalabial folds, and on the cheeks; key sign of this condition is the cluster pattern of the papules, occurring in little "groups"; occurs almost exclusively in women in their early 20s through their mid- to late 40s

**perioral rhytide**   wrinkles around the mouth

**pheomelanin (fee-oh-melanin)**   a red-yellow pigment found in red hair

**physical sunscreen ingredients**   work by reflecting or scattering rays from the skin

**pilosebaceous unit (pile-oh-seb-ay-shous)**   the entire structure of the follicle including the sebaceous glands

**poikiloderma of Cevattes (poy-kee-low-derma of seh-vahts)**   a symptom of severe cumulative sun damage characterized by dark splotchy hyperpigmented and distended capillaries and diffuse redness in a horseshoe pattern on the neck

**pomade acne**   closed comedones, pimples, and papules that appear around the hairline and on the forehead and are caused by the use of occlusive or comedogenic hair products, specifically hair waxes, scalp oils, some gels, some hairsprays, and other styling products

**pores**   the openings or orifices of the sebaceous follicles on the surface of the skin

**post-inflammatory hyperpigmentation**   also known as PIH; dark pigment splotches that develop from inflammation to the skin such as a pimple, a scrape, or minor injury

**psoralen (sore-ah-len)**   a drug used to treat psoriasis

**pustule**   an infected follicle filled with pus


# R

**re-epithelialization (ree-eh-pith-ee-lee-ah-zay-shun)**   the process in which the epidermis is regenerated after an injury or wound

**reactive oxygen species (ROS)** refers to the many different forms of free radicals that cause oxidation

**retention hyperkeratosis** hereditary tendency of acne-prone skin and oily skin types to not shed cells from the skin surface or from the lining of the follicle in the same way that normal skin does

**retinoids** derivatives of vitamin A

**retinol** natural form of vitamin A often used in skin care products for aging and sun-damaged skin

**rhinophyma (rhino-fimah)** the term used to describe the enlarged nose of rosacea caused by swelling of the nose and growth of the cartilage in the nose

**rhytides** medical term for skin wrinkling

**rosacea** a hereditary vascular disorder that results in diffuse redness, facial swelling, acne-like papules and pustules, distended capillaries, and, in some cases, enlargement of the nose

# S

**SPF** stands for sun protection factor; represented by a number that measures how long you can stay out in the skin without getting a sunburn

**sebaceous filaments** often called clogged pores, they are follicles impacted with solidified, oxidized sebum

**sebaceous glands** secrete (produce) sebum, a complex of oily and waxy components

**sebaceous hyperplasias** overgrown sebaceous glands that are pressing upwards on the tissue around the follicle, creating a ridge around the follicle opening

**seborrheic dermatitis** a common condition that is an inflammation of the sebaceous glands that results in inflamed, red, and flaky skin; typically occurs in oilier areas of the face, such as the nose, scalp, brows, ears, and T-zone

**seborrheic keratosis** a pileup of cells, indicative of cumulative sun damage, that appears in a patch-like, slightly raised lesion; they often look like gray or flesh-colored scabs, almost as if they are "stuck" on the skin surface

**sodium ascorbyl phosphate** ester form of vitamin C

**solar lentigines** hyperpigmented spots caused from sun exposure; sun freckles

**solar mottling** uneven pigment resulting in splotchy freckling due to cumulative sun damage

**solar rhytides** wrinkles caused from sun exposure

**squamous cell carcinomas**   form of common skin cancer in which the lesions tend to look like crusty bumps and can vary in size; usually raised

**stratum corneum**   the outermost layer in the epidermis; also called the horny layer

**stratum granulosum**   the layer within the epidermis where cells begin filling with keratin

**stratum spinosum**   second innermost layer within the epidermis, where keratinocytes begin their migration to the skin surface

**subcutaneous layer**   layer beneath the reticular dermis that contains thicker layers of fat to give the skin protection and to cushion the internal organs

**subjective symptoms**   symptoms that are felt, but not visible; examples are itching or stinging

**superficial peels**   light peels that only remove corneum cells from the epidermis; performed by licensed estheticians and also may be performed in dermatology or plastic surgery clinics; superficial peels do not peel beyond the surface cells and do not cause any blistering or bleeding

**surfactants**   ingredients that reduce the surface tension on the skin, allowing products to slip across the skin; also used as cleansing agents and detergents

# T

**T-zone**   the oily area down the middle of the face in combination skin

**telangiectasias (teh-lan-ject-ay-juz)**   dilated capillaries

**tinea versicolor (tin-eh-ah verse-ih-coh-ler)**   a fungus that causes white spots on usually tanned skin

**tocopherol or tocopheryl acetate (tah-cah-fur-all)**   vitamin E

**transepidermal water loss (TEWL)**   describes moisture escaping from the epidermis, causing skin dehydration

**triggers**   a term used to describe factors that cause sudden reddening of the facial skin from sudden increased blood flow in persons with rosacea

# U

**ultraviolet alpha (UVA)**   longer and deeper-penetrating sun rays believed to cause the most damage in terms of premature skin aging, elastosis, and wrinkling, as well as skin cancers

**ultraviolet beta (UVB)**   shorter sun rays that penetrate the epidermis to the basal layer; UVB rays cause sunburns and most common skin cancers

**urticaria (urt-ah-care-ee-ah)**   hives

**UV index**   a measurement formula meteorologists use to describe the day-by-day intensity of the sun.

# V

**vascular**   involving the blood circulation

**vascular growth factor**   a biochemical within the skin that triggers expansion and growth of new blood vessels

**vehicle**   spreading agent in a skin care or cosmetic product

**vitiligo (vit-eh-lie-go)**   a chronic condition, believed by some medical scientists to be an autoimmune disease, in which the skin loses the ability to make pigment

# W

**winter itch**   dry, itchy, and flaky skin, caused from low winter humidity and lack of lipids in the barrier function

# X

**xanthelasmas (zan-thah-laz-mahs)**   small skin pockets of cholesterol that appear as flat yellowish bumps often around the eyes

**xerosis (zer-oh-sis)**   the medical term for dry skin

# BIBLIOGRAPHY

## BIBLIOGRAPHY AND RECOMMENDED READING

Fulton, J. (1984). *Dr. Fulton's step-by-step program for clearing acne.* New York: Barnes and Noble Books.

Lees, M. (2007). *Skin care: Beyond the basics.* Albany, NY: Milady.

Leffell, D. (2000). *Total skin.* New York: Hyperion.

Michalun, N. (2009). *Skin care and cosmetic ingredients dictionary.* Albany, NY: Milady.

Pugliese, P. (2001). *Physiology of the skin II.* Carol Stream, IL: Allured Publishing.

Pugliese, P. (2005). *Advanced professional skin care.* Bernville, PA: The Topical Agent LLC.

Turkington, C., & Dover, J. (2007). *Skin deep.* New York: Facts on File.

## PERIODICALS FOR PROFESSIONALS

*American Spa*
One Park Avenue
New York, NY 10016
212-951-6600

*Cosmetic Dermatology*
7 Century Dr.
Parsippany, NJ 07054-4609
800-480-4851

*Dayspa*
7628 Densmore Ave.
Van Nuys, CA 91406-2042
818-782-7328

*Dermascope*
4402 Broadway Blvd., Ste. 14
Garland, TX  75043
800-961-3777

*Les Nouvelles Esthetiques—American Edition*
3929 Ponce de Leon
Coral Gables, FL  33134
800-471-0229

*PCI (Progressive Clinical Insights) Journal*
484 Spring Avenue
Ridgewood, NJ  07450-4624
201-670-4100

*Skin, Inc.*
336 Gunderson Dr., Suite A
Carol Stream, IL
630-653-2155

*Skin and Allergy News*
5635 Fishers Lane, Suite 6000
Rockville, MD  20852
877-524-9336